Writing-to-Learn

Curricular Strategies for Nursing and Other Disciplines

Gail P. Poirrier, DNS, RN

NLN Press • New York

Pub. No. 14-7238

This book is dedicated to educators who value and use the power of language and writing in teaching/learning.

Copyright © 1997
NLN Press
350 Hudson Street, New York, NY 10014

Library of Congress Cataloging-in-Publication Data

Poirrier, Gail P.
    Writing-to-learn / Gail P. Poirrier.
       p. cm.
    Includes bibliographical references and index.
    ISBN 0-88737-723-8
    1. English language—Rhetoric—Study and teaching. 2. English language—Technical English—Study and teaching.
3. Interdisciplinary approach in education. 4. Nursing—Authorship—Study and teaching. 5. Technical writing—Study and teaching.
I. Title.
PE1404.P57   1996
808'.042'07—dc21   96–39400
                                              CIP

This book was set in Bodoni by Publications Development Company, Crockett, Texas. The editor was Allan Graubard. The printer was Bookcrafters. The cover was designed by Lauren Stevens.

Printed in the United States of America.

CONTENTS

Contents

Contents

PREFACE

W hat do students learn? How do students learn? What should they learn? Can students critically think? Can students express their thinking in written format? Does writing assist students to learn and think? Such questions and more are at the heart of any faculty led evaluation of teaching/learning outcomes. With new outcome-based directions of accreditation criteria from professional and legal organizations and accountability demands from the general public, it became even more vital to pose and attempt to answer such questions. In our nursing program, for example, while curriculum and assessment were at the heart of the entire educational process, there was also need for a new focus on teaching and learning. As a result, the difficult but rewarding task of student learning outcome measurement began. Immediately, critical thinking, writing, communication, and student learning outcomes became significant buzz words. By 1990, and as a consequence of faculty deliberation, a major curricular innovation to assist students to achieve learning goals relevant to the practice of nursing was instituted: the writing-to-learn program. By 1996, six years later, it is still flourishing with much success to its credit.

Writing-to-learn strategies that reflect critical thinking and communication skills, professional growth, research, and classroom instruction have been incorporated across the nursing curriculum at the University of Southwestern Louisiana in a baccalaureate program consisting of approximately 1,400 nursing majors. Several faculties have engaged in evaluative and instructional research related to the implementation of such curricular strategies, all with positive results.

Student retention rates improved as well as overall class grades. Better student and faculty attitudes about writing surfaced. Faculty and student publications increased as well as collaborative research efforts among faculty. It is time to share these success stories and curricular implementations of writing-to-learn, so that other nursing programs and disciplines can benefit.

Even at interdisciplinary conferences where health science is one field among others, the success of the project has prompted widespread attention. Audiences want more information about the details of incorporating and implementing writing-to-learn in their curricula. Thus, the purposes of this book are:

1. To inform teachers why writing-to-learn is important to education, practice, and research
2. To detail how to incorporate writing-to-learn into the curriculum
3. To depict the design of a writing-to-learn intense course
4. To provide examples of how to incorporate writing-to-learn across the program of studies
5. To present a compilation of effective writing-to-learn strategies, so as to enhance communication, critical thinking, professional growth, research, and classroom instruction.

Although this book is written for college teachers in many disciplines, it does emphasize writing-to-learn across the *nursing* curriculum here at the University of Southwestern Louisiana. As a result, the book's primary audience includes faculty members in nursing and associated health disciplines; nonetheless, all content in this book is applicable to other disciplines. As a group, it seems, college teachers need a book to guide them in understanding and implementing writing-to-learn concepts within their curriculum. In this book, then, are many detailed effective writing-to-learn strategies for teachers to adapt to their own discipline's curriculum. It is expected that university writing labs and centers, Writing Across the Curriculum (WAC) programs, teachers assigned to teach writing intense courses, student teachers, and graduate assistants will all benefit from this book.

In his 1994 booklet, *Writing Across the Curriculum*, Dr. Art Young, a national leader in writing across the curriculum, suggests that writing is important for disciplines that have "unique cognitive and rhetorical practices, ones that may not be generalizable across disciplines, such as writing proofs in mathematics, patient histories in nursing, or ethnographies in anthropology." This book complements Dr. Young's statement. Disciplines must first build their own sound curricular writing strategies before collaborative writing efforts can benefit all students and faculty within the total university community. I want to thank Dr. Art Young for his letter of support and encouragement to write this book.

My special thanks go to Dr. Ann Dobie, Professor of English for her belief in writing across the curriculum and writing-to-learn, high standards, and willingness to collaborate with a health science-oriented colleague. Ann, I thank you for your consistent support of writing-to-learn research, expertise, and hours devoted to workshops and meetings that you gave to nursing faculty to help them with their various writing projects.

I'm most grateful to the Department of Baccalaureate Nursing faculty who have accepted my writing-to-learn ideas and for their creativity in developing and implementing their own within their nursing courses. You have created my research playground and made this book possible.

To my husband, Steve, I thank you for your belief in my abilities and your love and support. I know that you have heard writing-to-learn more than any human being should have to, yet you continue to listen and give positive strokes when needed. I also thank my children, Keith and Katherine, for their contribution to my personal and professional growth.

Preface

And for those who wish to do so, the readers of this book, please let me know what you think; I offer my assistance in guiding you with your writing-to-learn projects. Write your comments and questions to: Dr. Gail Poirrier, College of Nursing Baccalaureate Program, Southwestern Louisiana University, P.O. Drawer 43810, Lafayette, LA 70504-3810.

FOREWORD

*T*his book makes an important contribution to nursing education. This book was written by nursing educators and clinical practitioners, who have chosen to implement writing-to-learn strategies in their own courses and who have examined carefully the results of such strategies on their students' performance and on their own teaching effectiveness. This book is their remarkable story.

This story begins in 1990 at Southwestern Louisiana University, when the nursing faculty undertook to revise its curriculum and teaching practices to meet new accreditation criteria and to satisfy their own desire to educate nurses who are technically proficient, professionally able, and better prepared to be lifelong learners and contributors to the health and healing professions. When I visited their campus in the spring of 1993 to conduct writing-to-learn workshops for a group of interdisciplinary faculty, it was clear that the nursing faculty was far ahead of many of their colleagues in implementing key transformations in their curriculum. And now, as I read through this book, I am very much impressed with how far they have come. I believe that they are forging a new synthesis among professional/liberal/technical education, one that lays a sound basis for nursing education into the 21st century. Indeed, this book offers all disciplines a valuable model for educational change, a model that includes teaching philosophy, faculty development, curricular integration, performance standards, and the formative and summative assessment that leads to continuous improvement.

Gail P. Poirrier's introductory chapters provide a sound, theoretical context for implementing writing-to-learn in the nursing curriculum. They are full of practical, classroom-tested ideas that all teachers will find accessible and valuable. She understands how useful a tool writing-to-learn is for students learning the knowledge of a discipline and discovering what it means to be a professional in that discipline. Traditionally, writing in college is frequently used to test a student's mastery of a subject, but Professor Poirrier is very persuasive in recommending that teachers use writing to help students learn subject matter and then to apply that knowledge in clinical and interpersonal settings. She takes us through the entire process: planning, research, faculty participation, interdisciplinary cooperation, changes in individual classes, and changes across the curriculum. For example, we are shown, step-by-step, how to plan an introduction to the nursing course (Chapter 3), one that fosters "active learning" for students and "interactive teaching" for instructors. Thus, this book will be valuable to individual instructors seeking to transform their teaching and to program directors and their colleagues seeking to build a coherent curriculum that addresses the needs of their students and meets national accrediting criteria.

Numerous nursing professors at Southwestern Louisiana University contributed their classroom-based research on teaching to this volume, indicating how pervasively writing-to-learn is practiced throughout this curriculum. Specific suggestions are offered for using various writing-to-learn strategies: journal writing, freewriting, unsent letters, computer-supported writing, and professional articles meant for publication. Just as important, we get these authors reflections on their planning processes and their assessments of results. They model for us, in a variety of writing-intense courses at every level of the curriculum, the writing-to-learn approach. We see writing assignments designed to combine students' life experiences with their developing understanding of clinical knowledge and professional expectations. We see assignments designed to encourage critical thinking, cooperative learning, interpersonal understanding, ethical reflection, and effective communication. We see assignments that are central to individual course goals and nursing curriculum objectives and not just "add-on" assignments, what students call "busy work," that is, not central to the factual basics of the course. We also hear these teachers' evaluations of these assignments and how they might be improved in the future. These authors understand that the primary purpose of writing in their curriculum is not to help English faculty teach the skill of writing (as some faculty mistakenly assume), but to make better prepared and more capable nursing professionals.

Some scholars differentiate between "writing across the curriculum" (WAC) and "writing in the discipline" (WID). Briefly, WAC involves those writing activities that might be useful in all courses; they are helpful tools in the learning of all disciplines. WID, on the other hand, involves learning to write in a particular discipline or profession; it means possessing a knowledge of a discipline and its ways of doing things that only an "insider" knows. Ideally, a coherent baccalaureate curriculum should involve both WAC and WID. It should employ language as a lifelong tool for learning and employ the specialized discourse of a particular discipline, in this case, the nursing profession. The curriculum presented in this volume is writing-intense in both of these ways. Students experience writing-across-the-curriculum strategies, such as keeping a course journal or receiving constructive feedback on drafts of a formal paper, that are applicable to most every course at the university. However, students also experience writing-in-the-discipline projects that are unique to nursing, such as writing an article for publication in a nursing periodical (Chapter 5) and writing newspaper articles for the general public on health promotion and maintenance from the point of view of the nurse as "care giver, advocate, and health teacher" (Chapter 13).

The story this book tells, then, is one that will be valuable to all teachers and program administrators, and it will be particularly valuable for nursing educators. While it is full of practical teaching strategies and wise advice on subjects such as curriculum planning, faculty development, and outcomes assessment, a no less important purpose is to provoke thought and action, to inspire us to make a difference in our students' lives. As teachers and professionals, our most crucial obligation is to educate the talent who will replace us in the future. This book is a good guide and companion as we consider how best to meet this obligation.

ART YOUNG, PHD
Campbell Chair in Technical Communication
Professor of English and Professor of Engineering
Clemson University

CONTRIBUTING AUTHORS

Anne B. Broussard, RNC, DNS,
 FACCE
Associate Professor
Semester Coordinator, First
 Semester Junior Year
College of Nursing
University of Southwestern Louisiana

Paula Broussard, RN, MN
Assistant Professor
Semester Coordinator, First
 Semester Senior Year
College of Nursing
University of Southwestern Louisiana

Carolyn Delahoussaye, DNS, RN
Associate Professor
Coordinator Master of Science in
 Nursing Program
College of Nursing
University of Southwestern Louisiana

Dr. Ann B. Dobie, Ed.D.
Professor of English
Chair, University Writing Advisory
 Board
College of Liberal Arts
University of Southwestern Louisiana

Susan Gardner, PhD
Writing Coordinator for the Faculty
School of Nursing
Westminster College of Salt Lake City

Christine Hult, PhD
Professor
Assistant Department Head
Utah State University

Peggy McCabe, RN, MSN
Assistant Professor
Coordinator Learning Resource
 Center
College of Nursing
University of Southwestern
 Louisiana

Teresa Mumme Margaglio, MS, RN,
 CS-FNP, IBCLC
Pediatric Nurse Practitioner
Pediatric Associates of Lafayette
Lafayette, Louisiana

Zoe New, MSN, RN, CETN, CRRN
Instructor
College of Nursing
University of Southwestern
 Louisiana

Melinda Oberleitner, DNS, RN,
 OCN
Assistant Professor
Semester Coordinator, Second
 Semester Junior Year
College of Nursing
University of Southwestern
 Louisiana

Contributing Authors

Gail P. Poirrier, DNS, RN
Associate Professor
Department Head, Baccalaureate
　Nursing
College of Nursing
University of Southwestern
　Louisiana

Susan M. Randol, RN, MSN
Instructor
Semester Coordinator,
　Freshman/Sophomore Courses
College of Nursing
University of Southwestern
　Louisiana

Susan W. Reynolds, RN, MS
Instructor
College of Nursing
University of Southwestern
　Louisiana

Rosemary Rhodes, DNS, RN
Professor
Director of Undergraduate Studies
Department Chair, Adult Health
　Nursing
College of Nursing
University of South Alabama
　at Mobile

Janis G. Weber-Breaux, PhD, CFLE,
　CFCS
Assistant Professor
College of Applied Life Sciences
University of Southwestern
　Louisiana

Stephanie D. Wiggins, DNS, RN
Assistant Professor
College of Nursing
University of South Alabama
　at Mobile

Evelyn M. Wills, PhD, RN
Assistant Professor
College of Nursing
University of Southwestern
　Louisiana

Art Young, PhD
Campbell Chair in Technical
　Communication
Professor of English and Professor of
　Engineering
Clemson University

INTRODUCTION

*I*s there a relationship between writing ability, learning outcomes, and thinking skills? Many years ago, Piaget stated that one learned by doing (enactive), by depiction in an image (iconic), and by restatement in words (symbolic). Writing naturally embraces all of these ways of learning. The focus of writing programs must be on teaching and learning, so that students can utilize the written language to develop and communicate knowledge in and across every discipline (Young, 1994). Educators can assist students to learn specific content in any discipline by implementing writing-to-learn activities in the classroom. The examples presented in Chapters Five through Eighteen offer proof that writing improves thinking and assists students in achieving curriculum learning outcomes that are essential for application to practice.

As educators, we want out students to write well. Students in science and professional schools demonstrate a decline in writing ability between college admission and graduation (Allen, Bowers, & Diekelmann, 1989; Smit, 1991). This pattern begins at the elementary and secondary school levels. According to Applebee, Langer, Jenkins, Mullis, & Foertsch (1990), the National Assessment of Educational Progress (NAEP) that tests writing abilities in grades 4, 8, and 12 reports that "across the entire set of writing tasks administered, performance varied considerably. At grade 4, the percentage of adequate or better responses ranged from 9 to 47 percent across tasks; at grade 8, the range was from 14 to 51 percent; and at grade 12, it was from 24 to 56 percent" (p. 8). Some years earlier, Applebee (1981) also suggested that poor writing performance was a direct result of the fact that students did not engage in much writing and were not instructed on writing techniques. Unfortunately this is often the case at the college level. Smit (1991) reports that in most colleges and universities across the country students write very little and do so via reports, summaries, term papers, poems, or short stories that are usually graded according to the teacher's expectations, with little relationship to learning outcomes.

In order to help students improve their writing and thinking skills, it is imperative for educators to believe that the quality of student writing is directly related to academic and career success. Educators must pay closer attention to the kind of writing that they assign (Olds, 1990), and do so with an open attitude, more collaborative teacher/student relationships, partnerships in teaching/learning processes, closer attention to the relationship between teaching/learning and student outcomes assessment, increased involvement in meeting individual learning needs in the classroom, creativity, and a basic understanding of the differences between writing-to-learn and the traditional learning-to-write activities.

WRITING-TO-LEARN VERSUS LEARNING-TO-WRITE

The following assumptions, as interpreted by Allen, Bowers, and Diekelmann (1989), are representative of the traditional learning-to-write paradigm (Hairston, 1983): Students learn regardless of writing abilities; writing and thinking require different skills and should be taught separately; knowledge about the subject is necessary to write about it; writing is a sequential activity and thus mastery of all components, like paragraph construction, is needed in order to write; communication of what one knows is the major purpose of writing; and the instructor is the assumed audience for the students. Learning-to-write suggests that composition experts should teach writing and that after mastery of all components of writing (simple or complex) the student can transfer these skills to other content areas such as nursing.

In comparison, the writing-to-learn paradigm (Bazerman, 1981; Kinneavy, 1980; Odell, 1980) offers assistance to students who must acquire a complex knowledge base in order to function safely, efficiently, and effectively in today's real world. Assumptions of this paradigm include the following (Allen et al., 1989):

learning occurs through writing; writing and thinking skills are inseparable; writing is dialectical as opposed to sequential; knowledge and understanding are products of the writing process; learning and discovery are important purposes of writing, as is communication; and each discipline sets their own standards for writing. Students learn writing within their own discipline while writing for real audiences. In the writing-to-learn paradigm, the educator generally wants the writer to report what he or she already knows or to communicate what has been learned. For example, technical writing is often required by nurse educators through charting, care plans, or process recordings. As a result, the nursing student must present such knowledge in one of these acceptable written forms.

WRITING-TO-LEARN TECHNIQUES

Writing-to-learn activities can be selected and designed for students to enhance understanding of content and ability to think and make decisions in practice settings, such as clinical nursing, business, social service, and so on. According to Tchudi (1986), writing-to-learn activities do assist students with learning and have distinct characteristics: They are generally short, in-class and impromptu; written primarily for the benefit of the writer to clarify specific content, a situation, or a lived experience; and does not require extensive instructor feedback or response. Writing-to-learn activities also allow for writing to be showcased in the classroom as a means of learning and thinking.

The following are examples of writing intensive activities that apply to the writing-to-learn paradigm (Gere, 1985; Smit, 1991). All of these writing activities can be used to clarify content and to develop higher level conceptual thinking, so that decisions or conclusions can be made in practice settings. Any one or any combination of these activities are applicable to theory courses, learning laboratories (skills lab), and clinical experience settings or field experiences.

- *Journal writing* can be an extension of class notes; can focus on one topic or broadly on one's feelings; can provide a means for students to raise issues and concerns by summarizing what they have learned (Hahnemann, 1986).
- *Freewriting* allows students to write free associations to whatever comes into their minds in response to a reading, lecture, or discussion (Tchudi, 1986).
- *Microthemes or mini-essays* require students to write summaries, pose questions, work with data, and provide support for generalizations (Tchudi, 1986).
- *Admit and exit slips* allow students to focus on the specific class objectives and topics for the day (Gere, 1985); admit slips are like admission tickets to class; exit slips can be used to provide closure for learning by asking students to summarize what has taken place during class.
- *Dialectics* allow for written interchange that leads to the development of new ideas about a subject and provides the student with a sense of personal engagement with the subject (Arkle, 1985).
- *Brainstorming* collects, in writing, all ideas generated by an individual or group given a topic (Gere, 1985).
- *Focused writing* demands the writer to concentrate on a specific topic during timed nonstop writing and is akin to brainstorming (Gere, 1985).
- *Scenarios* require written responses to a "situation" in terms of what they (the student) would do in that situation based on course content (Troyka, 1996).
- *Quickwrites* demand a fast writing response during class or lab time about the "gist" of what has just been discussed (Troyka, 1996).

All of these writing-to-learn activities reinforce dialogue with others while developing writing skills as well as providing students experience in writing for a peer audience. Writing-to-learn activities, in contrast to the traditional paper writing method, remove the judgment call from the instructor and thus provide a positive approach to learning and writing. Writing-to-learn activities foster individual and group risk taking in writing and learning.

REFERENCES

Allen, D. G., Bowers, B., & Diekelmann, N. (1989). Writing to learn: A reconceptualization of thinking and writing in the nursing curriculum. *Journal of Nursing Education, 28*(1), 6–11.

Applebee, A. N. (1981). *Writing in the secondary school.* Urbana, IL: National Council of Teachers of English.

Applebee, A. N., Langer, J. A., Jenkins, L. B., Mullis, I. V. S., & Foertsch, M. A. (1990). *Learning to write in our nation's schools: Instruction and achievement in 1988 at grades 4, 8, and 12.* Princeton, NJ: The National Assessment of Educational Progress.

Arkle, S. (1985). Better writers, better thinkers. In A. Gere (Ed.), *Roots in the sawdust* (pp. 148–161). Urbana, IL: National Council of Teachers of English.

Bazerman, C. (1981). What written knowledge does: Three examples of academic discourse. *Philosophy of Social Science, 11*, 361–387.

Gere, A. (1985). Glossary. In A. Gere (Ed.), *Roots in the sawdust* (pp. 222–228). Urbana, IL: National Council of Teachers of English.

Hahnemann, B. (1986). Journal writing: A key to promoting critical thinking in nursing students. *Journal of Nursing Education, 25*(5), 213–215.

Hairston, M. (1983). The winds of change: Thomas Kuhn and the revolution in the teaching of writing. *Current Issues in Higher Education, 3*, 4–10.

Kinneavy, J. (1980). *A theory of discourse.* New York: Norton.

Odell, L. (1980). The process of writing and the process of learning. *College Composition and Communication, 31*, 42–50.

Olds, B. M. (1990). Does a writing program make a difference? A ten-year comparison of faculty attitudes about writing. *Writing Program Administration, 14*(1–2), 27–40.

Piaget, J. (1977). *The development of thought: Equilibration of cognitive structure.* New York: Viking.

Smit, D. W. (1991). Improving student writing. In *Exchange: Idea paper #25*, Kansas State University: Center for Faculty Evaluation & Development.

Tchudi, S. N. (1986). *Teaching writing in the content areas: College level.* New York: National Educational Association.

Troyka, L. Q. (1996). Writing across the curriculum: A practical guide. *Symposium, 2*(1), 6–7.

Young, A. (1994). *Writing across the curriculum.* Englewood Cliffs, NJ: Blair Press, Prentice-Hall.

Chapter One

WRITING-TO-LEARN

**IMPORTANT FOR EDUCATION,
PRACTICE, AND RESEARCH**

*T*he writing-to-learn paradigm reconceptualizes the relationship between critical thinking and writing processes as mutually dependent (Kinneavy, 1980). In recent years, new perspectives have viewed writing as an important method by which to develop thinking. Older views, of course, viewed writing as a more simple recording of thought (Allen, Bowers, & Diekelmann, 1989). Writing-to-learn is putting into words what the students already know and incorporating new information being studied in a curriculum (Forsman, 1985). Writing-to-learn enhances the development of critical thinking and conceptual clarity. According to Arkle (1985), better writers become better thinkers.

Certainly, critical thinking here is of paramount significance. Critical thinking, however, has been defined in many different ways. Paul (1990) refers to critical thinking as a disciplined, intellectual process of applying skillful reasoning as a guide to belief or action. Chaffee (1990) believes that critical thinking allows us to make sense of our work by enabling careful examination of the thinking process in order to clarify and improve understanding. Strader (1992) describes it as a process for examining underlying assumptions about current evidence and interpreting and evaluating arguments to reach a conclusion from a new perspective. Bandman and Bandman (1988) see it as the rational examination of ideas, inferences, assumptions, principles, arguments, conclusions, issues, statements, beliefs, and actions. Kozier, Erb, Blais, and Wilkinson (1995), state that *critical* means requiring careful judgment and *thinking* means having an opinion, reflecting, pondering, calling to mind, remembering, forming a mental picture, and reasoning; it is a purposeful mental activity in which ideas are produced and evaluated, plans made, and conclusions determined. Creative thinkers are also critical thinkers; both involve qualitative assessment and the production of new discovery (Paul & Bailin, 1988).

The National League for Nursing (1992) recognizes a critical thinking outcome as a specific criterion for the accreditation of baccalaureate programs. Nursing programs must include content and curricular activities designed to develop critical thinking skills. In practice settings, nurses use critical thinking to create new information and ideas, to make reliable observations, to draw sound conclusions, to evaluate lines of reasoning, and to improve their self-knowledge. "Thinking" precedes "doing" and nurses are engaged in a thinking-doing process daily, even hourly (Rubenfeld & Scheffer, 1995). Nurses rely on recall of their knowledge acquisitions, life experiences, capabilities of inquiry, creativity, intuition, and to generate new ideas to critically think before doing any aspect of nursing practice, such as assessing patients, diagnosing patient responses to illness, planning patient care, implementing patient care, and evaluating patient care outcomes. Nurses utilize Peterson and Stacks' (1994) four dimensions of critical thinking construct—factual, insightful, rational, and evaluative—in nursing practice. For example, nurses use *factual* thinking when they gather factual information and apply it to a given problem in a clear and precise manner. *Insightful* thinking is done routinely by nurses as they seek out possible goals and interpretations to given problems, which also fosters creative problem-solving skills. *Rational* thinking allows nurses to analyze logical connections among facts, goals, and assumptions relevant to a problem. When nurses use *evaluative* thinking, they reflect on value assumptions that underlie and affect decisions and interpretations that they and others make.

Writing-to-learn activities fit well within Peterson and Stacks' (1994) four dimensions of thinking construct that improve the capacity of people to learn, solve problems, and make decisions. A focused writing exercise can lead a student through a factual thinking process to make a decision about the most important information gained from the class topic of the day. This activity requires that the student write continually (nonstop) for five minutes explaining one important point about the day's topic. By pondering, sorting, and carefully judging the facts, the student forms an opinion and is able to extract important factual information from a large, complex content area. By examining all information given in class, the writing activity assists the student to engage in critical thinking by requiring the student to decide if the information considered important can be interpreted by others differently and if the key points are clear or ambiguous. Conceptual clarity here is important before students can apply decisions and actions based on concepts of any professional practice to given situations.

One exercise in particular, the unsent letter, assists the student to engage in insightful thinking. For example, the class topic—*trends, research, and politics*—introduces beginning clinical nursing students to standards of nursing practice and factors influencing nursing practice. Unsent letters are a form of role-playing that require students to write letters to someone under study or as a person involved in the material under discussion. Students could also be asked to think of a character who is a nurse in a movie, book, or television show. Based on the day's lecture and discussion, students are then asked to write a letter to the character, suggesting ways in which this character could more accurately represent a professional nurse. Twenty minutes is allocated to this exercise: ten minutes for actual writing and the other ten for sharing the letters in class. The student has to seek out a variety of interpretations that will lead to an alternate meaning or solution to improve the professional image of nursing. In order to be successful with this activity, the student must have some insights into his or her own thinking and understanding about the common, unprofessional public portrayal of nurses and how this one problem can impact on standards of practice, titling, licensing, and public policies that mandate nursing interventions and dictate reimbursement dollars for nursing services. This writing exercise assists the students to become better acquainted with nursing practice standards, public images of nurses in our society, consumer healthcare expectations of nursing practice, and the powerful impact of public communication on the current realities and future possibilities in nursing practice generally. The student critically thinks by rationally examining ideas, inferences, and principles as part of this role-playing writing-to-learn exercise. In addition, students share their writings with classmates and can critically think about different solutions to the problem.

Another exercise, writing the dramatic scenario, assists students to engage in rational and evaluative thinking. The instructor presents the students with a scenario (situation) that involves a legal/ethical conflict, such as an impaired nurse and compromised patient safety. Students are requested to respond in writing to the scenario presented. Ten minutes near the end of the class is allocated for the actual writing time. Written responses are collected by the instructor who then randomly selects several to share with the class for discussion and comment during the last ten minutes of class time. Student writings are returned at the next class meeting for feedback. This writing-to-learn activity allows the student to critically think by analyzing logical connections among the ethical/legal facts relevant to the problem and at the same time to generate and evaluate the implications that follow the actual decision or decisions. Students rationally think through the issues about which strategies would be more effective and which decision gives credence to a stronger argument or judgment call by them and others. The activity also leads the student to recognize and express in writing the value assumptions that underlie and affect decision making. Students must evaluate their own values and feelings in this problem-solving writing-to-learn activity and explore their own capacities to respect those who hold different views on the issue than they do. This dramatic scenario allows students to engage in a purposeful, reasoning mental activity in which ideas are produced, evaluated, and plans or decisions are made.

Students must find meaning in what they read for application to practice. Writing-to-learn techniques give students a personal connection with the material by allowing them to think on their own about the material (Gere, 1985). Writing and thinking skills are inseparable and necessary for discovery and critical understanding. With this new focus on evaluating critical thinking, educators must sharpen their expectations of students' writing skills and include specific writing-to-learn activities in the classroom. There is no better way to know how students think than to require students to explain themselves in writing. That writing skills can actually improve through critical thinking is also of some importance here

(Alfaro-LeFevre, 1995). As educators, we well understand that much of what students learn today will be obsolete tomorrow. As a result, we must aim at preparing students to be independent thinkers and to attend to learning that goes beyond assimilation of data.

As an enhancer of communication skills generally, writing-to-learn also helps students to gain knowledge and mastery of concepts and subject matter. Since writing-to-learn assists students to develop a better understanding of the subject matter and to critically think about what they have to say as they write, one can assume that this type of writing will be an effective means of communication for others. In this regard, when writing to communicate, Young (1994) finds due emphasis placed on the reading audience. The implication, of course, is clear: The writer has something to say and the reader wants to hear it and, in fact, takes the writer's ideas and opinions seriously. In order for this to happen, clarity of thinking and of communication is very important.

Nursing involves the use of many forms of written communication: reports, articles, policies, procedures, patient care notes, computerized charting, and so on. The written communication in practice should reflect the critical thinking skills associated with writing-to-learn and writing to communicate, including the self-conscious arranging, manipulating, and presenting of words and ideas that have been clarified for an audience to achieve a specific purpose (Young, 1994). Today, practitioners must be able to manage and use large volumes of scientific, technological, and patient information (PEW, 1991) to provide more cost efficient, effective, and integrated or coordinated healthcare to consumers. The healthcare system itself requires diverse communications skills from the skillful use of computer information systems to synthesize patient histories to the analysis of research findings to support the healthcare providers' treatment decisions based on outcomes, and to an ability to sort out and use valuable information to facilitate patient education, the patient becoming thereby an informed participant in decisions about his or her health care (de Tornyay, 1992). Nurses use clear communication skills, written and verbal, to:

1. Promote continuity and consistent quality care,
2. Provide evidence of critical thinking that accompanies the utilization of the nursing process,
3. Establish accountability for care, and
4. Develop nurse-patient and nurse-other health care provider relationships (Rubenfeld & Scheffer, 1995).

Research is essential to advancing nursing practice or any other discipline for outcome achievement. To advance research efforts educators must stay abreast of changes, identify gaps in the knowledge base, and initiate research projects (Rubenfeld & Scheffer, 1995). Writing-to-learn, which provides students with an opportunity to critically examine subject matter through writing, is an early introduction to the need to self-educate in relation to a discipline's knowledge base. Writing-to-learn activities assist students to clearly look at issues, explore alternative solutions to problems, and share ideas with peers and other audiences, important steps to "using research" in practice, and which the American Nurses Association (ANA, 1991) emphasizes as a standard of performance. Nurses are expected to use research findings whenever appropriate. Students can engage in writing research critiques as a means of "getting involved" in "using research" by exploring the literature and latest research findings and thinking about those findings in terms of clinical application.

REFERENCES

Alfaro-LeFevre, R. (1995). *Critical thinking in nursing: A practical approach.* Philadelphia: W. B. Saunders.

Allen, D. G., Bowers, B., & Diekelmann, N. (1989). Writing to learn: A reconceptualization of thinking and writing in the nursing curriculum. *Journal of Nursing Education, 28*(1), 6–11.

American Nurses Association. (1991). *Standards of clinical nursing practice.* Washington, DC: Author.

Arkle, S. (1985). Better writers, better thinkers. In A. Gere (Ed.), *Roots in the sawdust* (pp. 148–161). Urbana, IL: National Council of Teachers of English.

Bandman, E., & Bandman, B. (1988). *Critical thinking in nursing*. New York, New York: Appleton & Lange.

Chaffee, J. (1990). *Thinking critically* (3rd ed.). Houghton Mifflin.

de Tornyay, R. (1992). Reconsidering nursing education: The report of the PEW Health Professions Commission. *Journal of Nursing Education, 31*(7), 296–301.

Forsman, S. (1985). Writing to learn means learning to think. In A. Gere (Ed.), *Roots in the sawdust* (pp. 162–174). Urbana, IL: National Council of Teachers of English.

Gere, A. (1985). Glossary. In A. Gere (Ed.), *Roots in the sawdust* (pp. 222–228). Urbana, IL: National Council of Teachers of English.

Kinneavy, J. (1980). *A theory of discourse*. New York: Norton.

Kozier, B., Erb, G., Blais, K., & Wilkinson, W. (1995). *Fundamentals of nursing* (5th ed.). Lexington, MA: Addison-Wesley.

National League for Nursing. (1992). *Criteria and guidelines for the evaluation of baccalaureate and higher degree programs in nursing*. New York: Author. (Publication No. 15-2474)

Paul, R. (1990). *Critical thinking: What every person needs to survive in a rapidly changing world*. Center for Critical Thinking and Moral Critique, Sonoma State University, CA.

Paul, R., & Bailin, S. (1988). The creatively critical and critically creative thinker. In R. J. Marzano (Ed.), *Dimensions of thinking*. ERIC Clearinghouse.

Peterson, J., & Stacks, C. (1994). *The teaching for thinking project*. St. Paul, MN: Minnesota Community College System.

PEW Health Professions Commission. (1991). *Health America: Practitioner for 2005*. Durham, NC: Duke University Medical Center.

Rubenfeld, M. G., & Scheffer, B. K. (1995). *Critical thinking in nursing: An interactive approach*. Philadelphia: J. B. Lippincott.

Strader, M. (1992). Critical thinking. In E. J. Sullivan & P. J. Decker, (Eds.), *Effective management in nursing* (3rd ed.)(pp. 225–248). Lexington, MA: Addison-Wesley.

Young, A. (1994). *Writing across the curriculum*. Englewood Cliffs, NJ: Blair Press, Prentice-Hall.

Chapter Two

How to Incorporate Writing-to-Learn into a Curriculum

*W*riting-to-learn originates in and develops from a previous national curriculum movement known as Writing Across the Curriculum (WAC). Among other like curriculum movements, by introducing its agenda WAC has spawned several important interdisciplinary activities, especially enhancing faculty communication with faculty and, for our purposes here, promoting the incorporation of writing-to-learn in curricula to effect educational reform (Walvoord, 1996). At the curricular level, WAC has provided solutions to college students' lack of writing skills through the introduction of writing-to-learn strategies that focus on learning and aim at developing critical thinking and communication skills. The writing-to-learn approach addresses common interdisciplinary program goals that all college graduates be competent in written communication, be able to problem solve in their field of study, and be able to communicate processes and end results to society at large, which as we well know is composed of a multitude of different audiences. As a result, writing programs that adhere to the WAC agenda across curricula and disciplines have been successful. Reports (Bowers & McCarthy, 1993; Burling, 1982; Fulwiler & Young, 1990; Olds, 1990; Walvoord, 1996) indicate undergraduate development of analytic thinking skills, enhanced communication skills, increased valuing of writing skills by students, changed faculty attitudes and perceptions about learning and writing, and increased interdisciplinary communication.

The WAC movement blends well with new outcome-based directions of accreditation criteria as well. One purpose of accreditation is to foster continuous development and improvement in the quality of the educational programs (Tanner, 1993). Among WAC methodologies, writing-to-learn is specifically aimed at improving the quality of communication and thinking and thus improving the quality of learning within the educational process.

In terms of health care, which is currently undergoing dramatic change nationwide, both as a provider industry and an educational nexus, the latter needs are changing apace. PEW's third report (1995), for example, strongly recommends that nursing education examine its programs to better prepare a baccalaureate graduate to:

1. Function in an integrated system
2. Be more aware of diverse populations
3. Use resources
4. Be more innovative in the provision of nursing care or services
5. Be more inclusive in its definition of health
6. Be more concerned with education, prevention, and care management rather than treatment
7. Be more reliant on outcomes data and evidence.

In order to achieve PEW recommendations, nursing programs must also focus on outcome-based criteria (NLN, 1992) that relate to critical thinking, reasoning, research or decision making, communication, and interventions relevant to the discipline. Certainly, these same outcome-based criteria should be common across disciplines generally as well as being discipline focused.

WAC programs, which can activate much interest and enthusiasm among teachers, can also immediately produce interactive classrooms. With a focus on writing-to-learn, WAC offers the opportunity for all disciplines to meet quality education goals and accreditation criteria through the power of language, learning, interdisciplinary networking, and faculty empowerment.

University/Department Faculty: Winning Factors for Writing-to-Learn

Main resistance to incorporating writing-to-learn across a curriculum is the lack of university support for such projects and the misconception that the writing program will add faculty workload hours that lead to the wrong pathway for tenure and promotion.

University administrators are usually more receptive to writing programs if they can perceive an end result, such as enhanced administrative/faculty cooperation to effect needed educational changes that are in keeping with its mission statement.

Administrative support is essential for WAC programs to be successful. Administrators should appoint prestigious faculty members to oversee university-wide writing programs. These WAC committees must sell writing-to-learn programs as a positive means of improving learning and also educate faculty about the rewards in terms of teaching, professional activities, and research.

Disciplines beginning with writing-to-learn should seek the aid of WAC committees before initiating any pilot project. WAC committees can give consultation in terms of correctness, outcomes, techniques, networking opportunities with other on campus disciplines, implementation, and evaluation methods.

Prior to enlisting the help of a WAC committee, the leader (preferably the department head or curriculum chair) of the writing project must be sure the faculty are clear about writing-to-learn. Colleagues who work together for a common cause are generally more productive and serve as a self-motivating, powerful group for other faculty (Boice, 1992). The use of faculty strength is always a key factor to any curriculum reform. It is important to consider faculty autonomy when incorporating writing-to-learn into the curriculum. The individuality of the faculty involved in the writing project must be maintained in order to promote feelings of belonging and of being a worthy team member.

COLLABORATION FOR PLANNING AND IMPLEMENTATION

Begin incorporating writing-to-learn in the curriculum by assessing all current writing assignments. Assess each required course in the discipline and explore expectations related to writing and learning at each level of progression within the program. Closely examine the reasons for the current assignment and critically ask what the student will learn by this writing assignment. Also talk to currently enrolled students to better understand their views about writing within the curriculum. After assessment is complete, schedule an informal meeting with the chair of the WAC committee. Be prepared to discuss writing and learning as it applies to your specific curriculum, what type of writing is required by graduates of your program, and new ideas and directions related to writing and learning in your program of study.

Benefit from the experts in WAC and writing-to-learn. Self-educate as much as possible about writing-to-learn through workshops, literature reviews, networking with successful faculty and leaders of writing-to-learn across disciplines, and visits to other university programs. Explore writing centers and labs.

Choose a small group of faculty who support writing-to-learn and thoroughly educate this group about WAC and writing-to-learn. Send them to on-campus and national workshops where they can intellectually exchange ideas with colleagues from different disciplines. After attendance at workshops, meet with faculty on an individual basis to discuss their newly acquired knowledge and how to incorporate writing-to-learn within their specific course to advance student learning. Then introduce WAC and writing-to-learn to full faculty. A faculty meeting can become a workshop session. Invite the chair of the university WAC committee to do the presentation. Be sure that the previous small group of faculty already oriented to writing-to-learn is present and willing to act as mentors to the rest of the faculty. It is important at this meeting to assist the faculty to make connections between writing-to-learn strategies, outcomes, and research. Faculty need to hear that the rewards for incorporating writing-to-learn are realistic and obtainable. The implementation of writing-to-learn strategies can open new avenues for research related to student outcomes assessment. As educators, we must know if the strategy is worth repeating, if and what the student learned, how did the writing strategy help to achieve writing goals within the discipline, and how did the faculty benefit from their own efforts. Some examples of research questions to share with faculty during their writing-to-learn orientation include:

- How did writing strategies implemented in the writing intense course impact student grades?

- Did student attitudes toward writing change after the completion of a writing intense course?
- Are student retention rates better in courses that utilize writing-to-learn strategies?
- Does the writing-to-learn activity, clinical reasoning exams, increase critical thinking skills?
- Which writing-to-learn strategies best enhance communication skills?
- How does the writing-to-learn strategy, computer portfolio writings, enhance communication skills?
- Did faculty publications and research efforts increase as a result of individual faculty involvement with writing-to-learn activities?
- How does writing-to-learn curricular activities affect student perceptions of faculty caring?
- Does writing-to-learn assist teachers to be more outcome oriented?

After all faculty have been oriented, it is time to choose a starting place in the curriculum. There is no general rule to follow. The assessment of current writing in the curriculum, specific departmental writing goals and expected student outcomes, WAC's on-campus goal statement, and the mission of the university will help with this decision. Consider all benefits of writing-to-learn and research opportunities for faculty. The first pilot must be carefully planned. Assistance from the experts and the previously mentioned small faculty groups of mentors must be available for the individual faculty member(s) or groups of faculty implementing the writing project.

Developing a writing intense course (see Chapter Three) as a start really makes the incorporation of writing-to-learn meaningful and legitimate. Writing-intense courses allow the teacher to employ numerous writing-to-learn strategies. This in turn enriches the faculty member's understanding of the whole concept. At least 50 percent or more of the classes must use writing-to-learn activities to qualify as a writing-intense course. This takes planning time. Course unit objectives and the selected writing-to-learn activity have to connect. The specific learning outcome in keeping with the unit objective must be determined for each classroom writing activity. In-class time allocations for the writing activities need to be set. Questions regarding evaluation of student writings must be determined. An orientation to the writing project at the beginning of the class has to be planned for students.

Incorporation of writing-to-learn may begin with a single writing project in any required curriculum course. The activity should be designed for a single purpose, such as, enhancing learning, critical thinking, communication, research process, or professional development. Writing short critiques of intervention research for clinical practice or writing postcards about public policies to legislative groups are possible activities. Another approach is to implement writing-to-learn projects in several required curriculum courses at different educational levels, such as clinical reasoning exams which require students to respond to a situation by writing an essay (see Chapter Four). Writing-to-learn may be incorporated by expanding previous writing projects already in the curriculum at various levels. For example, nursing students at different educational levels may write a timed one-page belief statement about nursing and then share their writing with the class. This would replace the 2 to 3 page formal, philosophical paper generally written in the beginning courses. Across-the-curriculum implementation is not recommended at the start. Thorough evaluation and revision or modification of any new writing-to-learn project is necessary prior to total curriculum incorporation.

IMPLEMENTING WRITING-TO-LEARN
IN THE CURRICULUM

With detailed planning related to the actual writing-to-learn project, implementation of the project should be smooth. The implementation concerns are centered around instructor management of the writing-to-learn project within the context of the course and classroom environment. The success of the project is also dependent upon administrative involvement with particular attention to faculty workload and positive recognition of the faculty's commitment to the value of teaching for student learning. Essential steps to follow when implementing any writing-to-learn project include:

- Understand writing-to-learn.
- Understand the mission of the educational unit related to writing projects within the program.
- Identify expected student learning outcomes related to the writing project.
- Maintain open communication with unit administrators and WAC committee.
- Seek consultation from unit administrators, WAC committee members, and other experts.
- Invite administrators and WAC committee members to attend and evaluate classes periodically.
- Explain purpose of each writing-to-learn project and the evaluation method clearly to students.
- Discuss connection with specific learning objectives and specific writing-to-learn activities with students.
- Maintain notes relevant to strengths and weaknesses regarding in-class writing-to-learn activities.
- Adhere to planned time allocations for writing project.
- Share experiences with other faculty at meetings.
- Evaluate the student learning outcomes.
- Identify research possibilities.
- Modify, revise, and/or reject project.

Student learning outcomes dictate continuance of the writing project. If the initial pilot is successful, then expand to other courses. When the expansion includes different courses at various educational levels in the program, then brainstorm about incorporation across the total curriculum. At this point, writing-to-learn has been accepted by faculty as a positive method to improve student learning and writing skills.

References

Boice, R. (1992). *The new faculty member: Supporting and fostering professional development.* San Francisco: Jossey-Bass.

Bowers, B., & McCarthy, D. (1993). Developing analytic thinking skills in early undergraduate education. *Journal of Nursing Education, 32*(3), 107–114.

Burling, R. (1982). An upper-division writing course. *Southern Regional Education Board, 14*(1), 4–5.

Fulwiler, T., & Young, A. (1990). *Programs that work: Models and methods for writing across the curriculum.* Portsmouth, NH: Boynton/Cook.

National League for Nursing. (1992). *Criteria and guidelines for the evaluation of baccalaureate and higher degree programs in nursing.* New York: Author. (Publication No. 15-2474)

Olds, B. M. (1990). Does a writing program make a difference? A ten-year comparison of faculty attitudes about writing. *Writing Program Administration, 14*(1–2), 27–40.

PEW Health Professions Commission. (1995). *Critical challenges: Revitalizing the health professions for the twenty-first century.* San Francisco, CA: University of California at San Francisco, Center for the Health Professions.

Tanner, C. A. (1993). Thinking about critical thinking. *Journal of Nursing Education, 32*(3), 99–100.

Walvoord, B. E. (1996). The future of WAC. *College English, 58*(1), 58–79.

Chapter Three

DESIGNING A WRITING-TO-LEARN INTENSE COURSE

A writing-to-learn intense course provides students with a wide variety of writing activities in the classroom that directly relate to specific course objectives and the nature of the content being taught. Students learn writing within their own discipline while writing for real audiences in the classroom. Planned writing-to-learn exercises are integral components of every classroom presentation in designated courses. Such *writing-intense* courses foster higher order learning and aim at writing activities that enhance decision making, conceptual learning, and communication (Allen, Bowers, & Diekelmann, 1989).

COURSE SELECTION

Departmental acceptance of writing as a valuable learning tool is a must prior to choosing a starting place for the implementation of writing-to-learn concepts in any curriculum. Course selection should complement the faculty's commitment to seize upon the values of writing to enhance the critical thinking and communication skills of students. Courses that address real-life conceptual issues in the classroom make for easier design of a writing intense course. Examples of such courses include, but are not limited to, introduction to nursing, ethics and legal issues, gerontological nursing, cultural aspects of health, parenting, death and dying, and oncology nursing.

Choosing the introductory course as a writing-intense course has several advantages. A wide variety of writing-to-learn activities related to course objectives can be designed for each classroom presentation in an introductory nursing course. Introductory nursing courses generally introduce students to basic concepts that underlie nursing practice, professionalism, nursing roles, and health/illness issues. Thus, an introductory nursing course provides the setting for short, in-class freedom of expression writing that allows students to explore new concepts with other classmates and the instructor.

Since this is the first nursing course in most nursing curricula, students are introduced to writing-to-learn concepts at the beginning of their educational nursing experience. This sets the stage for establishment of writing expectations and standards within the discipline and creates an avenue for further curricular application of writing-to-learn principles.

Once the course selection has been made, the course description should reflect the writing-intense designation within the official records of the department and university catalog (Glick, 1988). This makes the departmental commitment to adopt writing-to-learn concepts official and creates new avenues for networking with university in-kind support services such as Writing Labs and Writing Across the Curriculum (WAC) programs.

FACULTY SELECTION

Assigning the "right" faculty to teach a writing-intense course is an important step toward success or failure of the project. The "right" faculty are flexible, innovative, knowledgeable, and open. The instructor must be flexible in utilizing new teaching methods in the classroom. Writing-to-learn activities are different for each classroom presentation. In the classroom setting, the instructor will use lecture presentations for dissemination of knowledge, use writing-to-learn application activities for higher level learning of the content, guide in-class discussions of the writings, and clarify content through utilization of the writing expressions and discussions. These teaching methods require the faculty to be creative and innovative in classroom leadership to move through the various transitions of teaching/learning in the daily classroom presentations and writing activities. It is a real challenge to actually lead an intense-writing class so that the higher order learning outcomes are achieved rather than just completing fragmented and meaningless writing sessions.

The instructor must be knowledgeable, not only in relation to the required course content, but about the writing-to-learn paradigm (Elbow, 1986). This knowledge base will enable the instructor to choose appropriate writing-to-learn activities in relation to content objectives and to be more open to cues from students during the total classroom experience.

Another factor to consider when selecting the "right" instructor to lead a writing-intense course is the individual's desire for professional growth in teaching and research. If the instructor has the motivation to learn more about the writing-to-learn concept for instructional research and development of new teaching methodologies, then that individual brings a strong commitment and desire for success of the project to the classroom setting.

When implementing writing-to-learn concepts in an introductory course, this instructor is the first contact in the educational program for the student. The instructor must be a positive role model who has the necessary teaching and management skills to be effective. This individual will lay the building blocks for future writing-to-learn curricular innovations, research, and scholarly activities.

COLLABORATION: IN-KIND SUPPORT

Seek interdisciplinary assistance at the beginning of the writing-intense course design. Members of Writing Across the Curriculum (WAC) committees, directors of writing labs, and English professors can provide technical information regarding appropriate writing-to-learn strategies, time allocations for specific writing assignments and clarity of course-specific writing outcomes (Young, 1994). These individuals or advocates of writing can present workshops that focus on writing-to-learn concepts and the technical details of writing-to-learn strategies such as timing, use in the classroom, evaluation, feedback, and appropriateness relevant to course content. Planning work sessions should be scheduled with the course instructor, department head and curriculum chair, and the writing-to-learn expert to actually design the writing intense course. This form of professional communication can set the framework for collaborative models across university curricula and strengthen the goals of WAC programs within the university setting. Future interdisciplinary partnerships for innovations in instruction, improvements in teaching/learning modalities, and ongoing research can result.

LINKING WRITING-TO-LEARN STRATEGIES TO COURSE OBJECTIVES

Students respond favorably to an open classroom environment, one that allows self-expression and sensory stimulation. Faculty need to recognize self-expression as relevant learning when content is being studied. Students respect activities that demand their attention to course material. For example, students are more attentive to films when one has to write key points after the viewing (Stevens, 1985). Students also value learning when they can see its relevance to what they already know and connect to their past life experiences. Faculty need to include exploration of such connections as part of instructional units and specific course objectives. Learner objectives provide the basis for evaluating whether learning has taken place (Kozier, Erb, Blais, & Wilkinson, 1995). Writing-to-learn activities should be developed to enhance the nature of the content being taught while complementing the course objectives for the promotion of learning (Allen, Bowers, & Diekelmann, 1989).

In an introductory nursing course, conceptual topics generally presented include introduction to nursing, socialization and roles, nursing trends, theories of nursing, healthcare delivery systems, health and illness, nursing process, stress and adaptation, grief, loss, and death. Selected writing-to-learn activities should focus on the course unit objectives for specific topics. Effective writing-to-learn strategies for previously mentioned topics include but are not limited to focused writings, admit and exit slips, buddy exchanges, unsent letters, microthemes, responses to dramatic scenarios, and problem-solution explorations (Gere, 1985). More specifically, when presenting the conceptual topic of grief, loss, and death, a unit course objective might be to discuss assisting patients to die with dignity. Directing students to engage in a focused writing activity (Gere, 1985), a timed paragraph explaining the meaning of dying with dignity and then sharing with the class, would be an appropriate writing-to-learn strategy designed to help the student achieve the unit objective and better comprehend the concept of grief, loss, and death. Another objective might be to describe Kübler-Ross's stages of grieving. To address this objective, students could be asked to write an unsent letter (Gere, 1985), a form of role-playing, to a family member or significant other describing their own grief process related to a personal loss. Both examples incorporate new knowledge, promote development of a more complex understanding of the conceptual topic, and address different audiences through writing.

EXAMPLES OF A WRITING-TO-LEARN INTENSE INTRODUCTORY NURSING COURSE

In 1992, the Department of Baccalaureate Nursing revised its introductory nursing course to reflect the concepts behind the Writing Across the Curriculum movement. The course was a writing-intense course designed to help students better understand the introductory nursing content through writing. The purpose was to assist students to grasp, integrate, articulate, think, and problem solve. Writing was the means by which students would engage in collaborative learning through peer critiques, sharing ideas and thinking, discussing writings, growing intellectually, and sharpening their critical decision-making skills.

Initially the writing-to-learn activities were planned for half of the class presentations. The writing sessions were short (ten to twenty minutes per class period), directly related to unit objectives, not graded, nonpunitive, and provided for constructive criticism of specific content or conceptual understanding. The pilot course was a success. Students verbalized that they wanted more writing.

Today, writing-to-learn activities are planned for each class presentation in the introductory nursing course. All student writings are collected by the instructor and returned at the next class meeting for constructive feedback (Smit, 1991). The focus of the feedback is understanding the nursing content being taught. If students demonstrate difficulties with use of grammar, spelling, poor sentence structure, and so on, a general comment directs students to assume responsibility to correct their difficulties. Five percent of the final course grade is based on writing participation by the individual student.

At our school, the same instructor teaches both sections of the introductory nursing course. Due to the large numbers of students (approximately 70 students per section) enrolled in the class, a clinical nursing instructor assists the classroom instructor in providing written feedback on all student writings. A 20 percent teaching workload is assigned for this assistance with the writing-intense course activities.

The following is a sample of the introductory course syllabus (Broussard, 1995) emphasizing the writing activities:

Nurs 114: Introduction to Basic Concepts in Nursing Course Description

Comprehensive introduction to nursing focusing on characteristics of the nurse, past and currently expanding roles, current health-care trends, and professional involvement. It is designed to present nursing as a humanistic, caring discipline focused on human beings and their health. The nursing process is introduced as a framework relating such concepts as exploration of human needs, dynamic nature of the wellness/illness continuum, adaptation, homeostasis, and sociocultural factors influencing the environment. Integrated intensive writing exercises assist the student in the synthesis of course content and concepts.

Topic I: Course Orientation

During the first class session, the course syllabus is reviewed in depth regarding major concepts and curricular themes, objectives, textbooks, interim advising, student-related policies, writing-intense exercises, and grading and evaluation. At the end of the orientation to the course, the instructor introduces the first in-class writing exercise designed to give students a "real" feel for writing-intense activities and in turn, information for the instructor to become more acquainted with the individual student. Students are asked to write short answers to several questions posed by the instructor. The following questions help students focus on the course design and purpose:

1. In five sentences or less, explain why you want to be a nurse?
2. Write, using complete sentences, at least three personal goals that you wish to achieve in relation to this course.
3. Do you think that writing is essential to success? Explain your answer in five sentences or less.
4. Briefly explain why you like or don't like to write.

Topic II: Introduction to Nursing: Socialization and Roles of the Nurse

Unit Objectives:

1. Identify the essential aspects which help to define nursing.
2. Discuss the historical development of nursing.
3. Explain professional growth within nursing.
4. Describe the five behaviors of the professional nurse as described by Miller.
5. Identify the critical components of professionalism.
6. Describe the roles of a professional nurse.
7. Discuss expanded roles of nurses.
8. Explain the functions of the various national nurses' associations.

Topical Outline of Content:
   A. An Emerging Definition of Nursing
   B. Significant Events in Nursing History
   C. Growth of Professionalism
   D. Process of Socialization
   E. Roles of the Professional Nurse
   F. Nursing Organizations

Teaching/Learning Strategies:
   Lecture/discussion
   Writing-intense exercise

Students are asked at the start of the class period to write an admit slip designed to assist students to focus their thinking on the assigned topic of the day or upcoming class discussion (Gere, 1985). The specific exercise requires students to write two separate paragraphs that complete the following phrases: "Nursing is . . .." and "In 5 years, my typical work day will be . . .". The writing exercise is limited to 10 minutes of classroom time. These writings not only assist the student to focus on topical content but gives the instructor an awareness of students' misunderstanding or confusion related to the content. This writing exercise will be repeated at the last class meeting of the semester, assisting students and faculty to examine individual growth and development related to defining and understanding what nursing is really all about.

Topic III: Trends, Research, and Politics

Unit Objectives:

1. Describe the recipients of nursing.
2. Identify the setting and focus of nursing practice.
3. Describe the standards of nursing practice.
4. Identify factors influencing nursing practice.
5. Explain how nursing education affects nursing practice.
6. Discuss the education, titling, and licensure of registered nurses.
7. Discuss the importance of continuing education in professional nursing.
8. Describe the role of nursing research as it influences current and future nursing practice.
9. Describe future trends in nursing.

Topical Outline of Content:
   A. Nursing Practice
   B. Nurse Practice Acts
   C. Standards of Clinical Nursing Practice
   D. Factors Influencing Nursing practice
   E. Nursing Education

F. Nursing Research

G. Future Trends in Nursing

Teaching/Learning Strategies:

Lecture/discussion

Writing-intense exercise

At the end of the class session, students are asked to write an unsent letter (Gere, 1985). Unsent letters are a form of role-playing that requires students to write letters to someone under study or as a person involved in the material under discussion. For this exercise, students are to think of a character who is a nurse in a television show. Then, based on the day's lecture and discussion, students are asked to write a letter to the writer, suggesting ways in which this character could more accurately represent a professional nurse. Twenty minutes is allocated to this exercise, ten minutes for actual writing and the other ten minutes for sharing the letters with the class. The instructor collects the letters and randomly reads several for brief in-class discussion. Letters, with instructor comments, are returned to individual students at the next class meeting. This writing exercise assists the students to become better acquainted with nursing practice standards, public images of nurses in our society, consumer healthcare expectations of nursing practice, and the powerful impact of public communication on current and future nursing practice in our society.

Topic IV: Theories and Conceptual Frameworks

Unit Objectives

1. Discuss the purpose of nursing theory.
2. Define the following terms: concept, conceptual framework, proposition, theory, construct, and hypotheses.
3. Identify common themes among selected nursing theorists.
4. Differentiate among general theorists, systems theorists, and interpersonal/caring theorists.
5. List the seven major units of a conceptual model of nursing.

6. Describe the relationship of nursing theories to the nursing process.
7. Discuss the USL College of Nursing Philosophy and Concepts.

Topical Outline of Content:
   A. Nursing Theories and Conceptual Models
   B. Overview of Selected Nursing Theories
   C. Major Units of Nursing Models
   D. Relationships of Theories to the Nursing Process
   E. USL College of Nursing Philosophy and Concepts

Teaching/Learning Strategies:
   Lecture/discussion
   Writing-intense exercise

This exercise requires each student to identify one major question regarding the topic of the day at the end of class time. Students are then instructed to state the question in writing and exchange the question with their "buddy" or classmate. The buddy's question is to be taken home and answered in writing. The answers and questions are collected at the next class meeting by the instructor for constructive feedback to the writer of the individual question. Five minutes of class time is utilized for the exchange. Buddy exchanges (Gere, 1985) usually begin with a statement of an opinion, a problem, a general misunderstanding or confusion regarding course material. The outcomes take the form of letters written to and from classmates. These serve as written dialogue between students about the course material and assist students to clarify course content.

Topic V: Healthcare Delivery Systems

Unit Objectives:

1. Define healthcare system.
2. Differentiate among primary, secondary, and tertiary healthcare delivery services.
3. Discuss the AHA Bill of Rights.
4. Identify the four types of healthcare delivery services.

5. Compare various healthcare agencies.

6. Discuss current issues and problems in healthcare delivery.

7. Summarize ANA recommendations for healthcare.

Topical Outline of Content:

    A. Rights of Healthcare

    B. Types of Healthcare Services

    C. Providers of Healthcare

    D. Healthcare Agencies

    E. Issues and Problems in Healthcare Delivery

    F. Nursing's Agenda for Healthcare Reform

Teaching/Learning Strategies:

Lecture/discussion

Writing-intense exercise

The same buddy exchange exercise utilized for the topic, *Theories and Conceptual Frameworks*, is repeated at this class session.

Topic VI: Introduction to Nursing Process

Unit Objectives:

1. Describe the components of the nursing process.

2. List benefits of the nursing process.

3. Discuss the nursing process as it relates to accountability and responsibility.

Topical Outline of Content:

    A. Evolution of the Nursing Process

    B. Components and Purposes

    C. Benefits

    D. Framework for Accountability

Teaching/Learning Strategies:

Lecture/discussion

Writing-intense exercise

The exit slip (Gere, 1985), a brief response written at the end of class time asking students to summarize what has been covered in class for that particular day, is utilized for the nursing process topic. Students are requested to write a short paragraph that summarizes the steps of the nursing process and explains why the nursing process is the basis for nursing practice. This exercise is allocated ten minutes in-class time.

Topic VII: Ethical and Legal Issues in Nursing

Unit Objectives:

1. Define ethics, values, and morality.
2. Discuss values and values clarification.
3. Discuss sources of ethical problems in nursing practice.
4. Identify factors which affect ethical decisions.
5. Describe general legal concepts as they apply to nursing.
6. Identify legal issues and areas of potential liability in nursing.
7. Discuss nurse practice acts.
8. Discuss the ICN and ANA codes of ethics.

Topical Outline of Content:
   A. Ethics, Value, and Morality
   B. Nursing Ethics
   C. Types of ethical problems
   D. Decision-making models
   E. Ethical issues in nursing practice
   F. Legal Concepts
   G. Liability
   H. Legal Responsibilities

Teaching/Learning Strategies:
   Lecture/discussion
   Writing-intense exercise

The dramatic scenario (Gere, 1985) exercise is most applicable to this topic. This writing exercise assists students to become involved in thinking through the issue(s). The instructor presents the students with a scenario (situation) that involves a legal/ethical conflict (code/no code procedures). Students are requested to respond in writing to the scenario presented. The writing time allocation is ten minutes at the end of the class. Written responses are collected by the instructor who then randomly selects several to share with the class for discussion and comment during the last ten minutes of class time. Student writings are returned at the next class meeting for feedback purposes.

Topic VIII: Wellness, Health, and Illness

Unit Objectives:

1. Define health, wellness, and well-being.
2. Explain the health/illness continuum.
3. Discuss variables that influence health status, beliefs, and practices.
4. Define illness and disease.
5. Describe illness behaviors.
6. Describe the nursing role in promoting health and wellness.

Topical Outline of Content:

    A. Concepts of health, wellness, and well-being

    B. Models of Health and Wellness

    C. Variables Influencing Health Status, Beliefs, and Practices

    D. Illness and Disease

    E. Health Promotion

Teaching/Learning Strategies:

    Lecture/discussion

    Writing-intense exercise

During the last ten minutes of class, students utilize exit slips (Gere, 1985) to write a summarized description of their family's health based on the components of the day's topic. This exercise allows students to better comprehend health and illness concepts through introspection.

Topic IX: Promoting Wellness Through the Lifespan

Unit Objectives:

1. Describe essential facts related to growth and development.
2. Explain the principles of growth and development.
3. Discuss application of principles of growth and development to nursing practice.
4. Identify age-related components of the USL College of Nursing Philosophy.

Content Outline:
   A. Factors Influencing Growth and Development
   B. Application of growth and development concepts to nursing practice
   C. Age-related concepts: USL CON philosophy

Teaching/Learning Strategies:
   Lecture/discussion
   Writing-intense exercise

Students are asked to engage in a focused writing exercise (Gere, 1985) at the end of the class, explaining one important point about the day's topic. The instructor directs students to write continually (nonstop) for five minutes about their chosen point of interest related to the lecture discussion for the day. This exercise assists students to concentrate and extract important factual information from large content areas.

Topic X: Stress and Coping

Unit Objectives:

1. Discuss the concepts of stress.
2. List physiological, cognitive, and psychological manifestations of stress.
3. Discuss modes of adaptation.

4. Describe characteristics of adaptive responses.

5. Discuss mechanisms for stress management.

6. Identify sources of stress in nursing.

Topical Outline of Content

    A. Concepts of Stress

    B. Manifestations of Stress

    C. Adaptation

    D. Nurse Management of Stress

Teaching/Learning Strategies:

    Lecture/discussion

    Writing-intense exercise

For this exercise, students are directed to use a dialectical format (Gere, 1985). Students are asked to divide a page of writing paper in half. On one side, students take notes on readings or lecture material; the other half is reserved for personal responses, questions, analysis comments, etc. This exercise assists students to cue important aspects of the topic and to prepare notes for later study. Students are asked to describe a stressful and difficult situation encountered in their life on the left side of the writing page. Directly opposite on the right side of the writing page, students are to explain how one coping strategy discussed in class today would apply to their situation. This is a ten minute exercise at the end of class.

Topic XI: Loss, Grieving, and Death

Unit Objectives:

1. Define loss and grief, and death.

2. Discuss loss as crisis.

3. Describe Kubler-Ross's stages of grieving.

4. Discuss assessment of the grieving patient.

5. Discuss assisting patients to "die with dignity."

Topical Outline of Content:

    A. Loss

    B. Crisis

    C. Grief

    D. Dying

    E. Needs of the Dying Client and the Family

Teaching/Learning Strategies:

    Lecture/discussion

    Writing-intense exercise

Students are directed to write as many negative statements about death and dying as possible in a five-minute, nonstop writing session at the start of the class session. This free writing exercise (Smit, 1991) at the start of class assists students to explore many characteristics of death and dying. During the class session, some of their written statements may be within the context of the instructor's lecture which assists students to make a better connection with the course material.

KEY POINTS IN IMPLEMENTATION AND EVALUATION

At the start of a writing-intense course, students must be oriented to the writing-to-learn concept. It is imperative for students to understand the purpose of each writing-to-learn strategy in relation to course objectives and conceptual content. Students need to be shown from the start that these in-class writing activities are designed to help with their understanding of content, enhance their critical thinking, communication skills, and problem solving in practice settings. Actually, students will "feel" the writing process and make connections between reading, writing, thinking, and learning while engaging in short, purposeful, in-class writing activities. In addition, students will verbally communicate their writing to a peer audience in many of these activities. This provides valuable feedback which assists the students in recognizing their own level of understanding.

Teaching a writing-intense course can be time consuming. Writing-to-learn activities must be meaningful in terms of course objectives. These activities require planning and are not easy to implement. The instructor must be able to lead the class from lecture to writing then back to lecture and perhaps more writing activities within the assigned time limits of the course. Special consideration must be given to time allocations for writing activities. The writing activities should provide for active learning and should never be interpreted by students as a punitive process (Glick, 1988).

Feedback is essential for learning. Someone should read the writings and give constructive feedback relevant to course objectives and content (Smit, 1991). Instructors will need to read certain writings while peers or classmates will read and respond to others. Some writing-to-learn activities may require the instructor to randomly read the writings to the class to further clarify a topic or concept. Feedback should focus on understanding of content and not correct use of grammar or spelling. If the later are problematic, then the instructor should inform the student so that the student accepts the responsibility to improve in those areas. It may be necessary to refer students to university writing centers for technical writing assistance.

An instructor may choose to grade or not grade the writings. Grading can be a hindrance to future writing in some cases. However, students need to be held accountable in terms of participating in the classroom writing activities (Young, 1994). Some type of reward system, like bonus points toward the final course grade, would be a positive strategy.

Large classes pose a great challenge to the idea of writing-intense courses. However, writing-to-learn activities can be developed for use in large classes as well as small. Group writings and increased use of peer exchange in the classroom are helpful when implementing in large classes. Checklists are also helpful to assist instructors to pinpoint the relevant points in certain writings for feedback purposes (Allen, Bowers, & Diekelmann, 1989). Other instructors can be assigned to assist the primary instructor to provide necessary feedback to student writings.

RESEARCH OPPORTUNITIES

Designing and implementing writing-intense courses gives the faculty member much opportunity to acquire new knowledge and creates a natural path to the research process. The writing-to-learn strategies introduce faculty to new teaching methodologies that serve as a basis for scientific inquiry. Instructional research investigations can determine if writing-to-learn strategies are effective in enhancing critical thinking, communication skills, and conceptual learning. Improved learning is an outcome of writing-intense courses. Studies could be aimed at comparing retention outcomes in writing-intense versus nonwriting-intense courses.

Students enter writing-intense courses with certain values and attitudes about writing in general. Researchers could develop measuring tools or instruments designed to test the effects of writing-intense strategies on student attitudes about writing. Tool development of this nature paves the way for faculty to use multiple approaches and methods, qualitative or quantitative, in instructional research. Such research studies could strengthen the writing-to-learn paradigm, improve instructional methods, and foster more evaluative research efforts.

The incorporation of writing-to-learn across a curriculum can provide important data for outcome assessment and program evaluation. This data can assist programs to better assess and evaluate student outcomes in critical thinking and communication and to plan new strategies for necessary program or curricular changes.

Writing-to-learn strategies can be utilized by any discipline. Writing-intense courses can be collaborative ventures among disciplines. Capstone courses that address common cross-discipline concepts like problem-solving and communication concepts are good examples (Olds, 1990). Cross-disciplinary writing-to-learn projects combine the skills of several faculty using linked or paired courses in which students take a writing course along with a course in another discipline and the faculty collaborate in teaching. Finally, disciplines have a common thread in the classrooms. This commonality serves as a vehicle for interdisciplinary research efforts. Collaborative research of this nature could foster uniformity to improve the quality of instruction and the image of the university across the whole campus.

REFERENCES

Allen, D. G., Bowers, B., & Diekelmann, N. (1989). Writing to learn: A reconceptualization of thinking and writing in the nursing curriculum. *Journal of Nursing Education, 28*(1), 6–11.

Broussard, P. (1995). *Unpublished syllabus: Department of Baccalaureate Nursing.* Lafayette, LA: University of Southwestern Louisiana.

Elbow, P. (1986). *Embracing contraries—Explorations in learning and teaching.* New York: Oxford University Press.

Gere, A. (1985). Glossary. In A. Gere (Ed.), *Roots in the sawdust* (pp. 222–228). Urbana, IL: National Council of Teachers of English.

Glick, M. D. (1988). Writing across the Curriculum: A dean's perspective. *WPA: Writing Program Administration, 11*(3), 53–58.

Kozier, B., Erb, G., Blais, K., & Wilkinson, J. M. (1995). *Fundamentals of nursing: Concepts, process, and practice* (5th ed.). Lexington, MA: Addison-Wesley.

Olds, B. M. (1990). Does a writing program make a difference? A ten-year comparison of faculty attitudes about writing. *Writing Program Administration, 14*(1–2), 27–40.

Smit, D. W. (1991). Improving student writing. In *Exchange: Idea paper #25.* Kansas State University: Center for Faculty Evaluation & Development.

Stevens, R. S., III. (1985). Writing and learning: What the students say. In A. Gere (Ed.), *Roots in the sawdust* (pp. 211–221). Urbana, IL: National Council of Teachers of English.

Young, A. (1994). *Writing across the curriculum.* Englewood Cliffs, NJ: Blair Press, Prentice-Hall.

Chapter Four

INCORPORATING WRITING-TO-LEARN ACROSS THE CURRICULUM

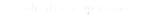

*C*hapter Two discusses planning and implementing writing-to-learn in the curriculum and lists essential steps to follow when implementing any writing-to-learn course in the curriculum. In this chapter, we consider terminal or graduate objectives that must be considered and connected with the writing project.

For across-the-curriculum incorporation of writing-to-learn, student learning outcomes should be identified for various levels while maintaining specific and unique writing exercises that truly complement certain courses in the curriculum. For example, journal writing complements student analysis of maternal/child bonding and family relationships in an obstetrics nursing course. When using themes related to learning outcomes across the curriculum, other writing projects may address professional development, critical thinking, and communication. This "theme" method of across-the-curriculum incorporation of writing-to-learn addresses both course specific and terminal or graduate objectives of the discipline. Writing exercises flow from simple to complex, from parts to whole, and are standardized within the curriculum. This allows for easier orientation of new faculty. The educational unit becomes unique with ready data for outcomes assessment, research, accreditation, and other reports.

Across-the-curriculum incorporation requires full faculty involvement. These strategies meet the student learning needs as well as the research and professional needs of the faculty. Keep in mind the research and professional growth opportunities associated with writing-to-learn curricular activities. Examples of writing-to-learn strategies that can be implemented across the curriculum follow.

First nursing courses in baccalaureate programs generally introduce nursing students to nursing roles, professionalism, health/illness issues, death and dying, nursing process, and other concepts that underlie nursing practice. The across-the-curriculum theme at this level addresses writing for knowledge acquisition, learning, and professional growth. The writing-to-learn strategy that works well at this level in baccalaureate nursing is an intense writing course. As mentioned in Chapter Three, introductory courses are great settings for intense writing courses. Various writing assignments are designed to connect with each class topic and provide short, in-class exercises that allow students to explore the new concepts of nursing with other classmates and the teacher. For example, key words from course unit objectives spark a focused writing experience for students by having them explain the meaning of a newly introduced nursing concept (i.e., the advocacy role) in a timed, written paragraph and then sharing their thoughts with the class. One important aspect of writing-to-learn instructional activities is the reinforcement of dialogue with others in developing these writings as well as providing students experience in writing for a peer audience. The exercises are not graded but require feedback from the instructor.

As students progress from introductory nursing courses to more advanced clinical courses, writing activities should focus on the theme of writing to enhance critical thinking skills. Writing-to-learn strategies should assist students in developing higher level thinking skills that will enhance clinical decision making. The clinical reasoning exam, for example, presents a hypothetical clinical situation. Students respond to the questions related to the situation. Questions should elicit critical thinking relevant to application of the nursing process and be designed so that there are no exact or absolute correct answers. The situations should reflect the knowledge relevant to the specific clinical course (child care, maternal/infant care, community mental health, and adult health) and give rise to a broad range of questions that relate to knowledge about disease processes, treatment regimens, nursing interventions, assessment data, community resources, discharge planning, clinical research, and ethical/legal issues. If the clinical courses are sequential, then the clinical reasoning exams need to be planned across the curriculum so that higher order testing can occur between the clinical nursing courses. Critical thinking is one of the required outcomes of nursing education (NLN, 1992).

Grading is recommended because this written exam measures the student's skills in reasoning, analysis, and decision making relevant to the discipline of nursing.

Critical thinking depends on mutual exchange of ideas. Another writing-across-the-curriculum theme is writing to improve communication skills. Communication is another required outcome of nursing education (NLN, 1992). Writing-to-learn activities aimed at enhancing communication skills can occur in any required course. Junior and senior level core concept courses that focus on communication skills, including use of computers in nursing and ethical/legal/moral issues are great for these writing strategies.

Students could be asked to write healthcare instructions for a complex wound-care procedure to be done in the home. Group writing assignments, such as case studies or analysis of nursing interventions and patient outcomes, facilitate group process learning and enhance communication and thinking skills by each group member engaging in a dialogue with self and others (Bruffee, 1978). Require students to write postcards to legislators expressing support of a needed change in public policy that affects elder healthcare. Students could write about a health promotion topic for a local newspaper, such as communicating the bad effects of the sun on the skin to the general public.

Sophomore through senior level students might be required to maintain a computer portfolio that contains printouts of various assignments relevant to the semester courses in which enrolled (see Chapter Ten). These assignments can vary from care plans, literary computer searches, E-mail messages, resumes, reports, critiques, and so on. The portfolio shows evidence that nursing students can write for communication purposes by utilizing computer technology. Students can write care plans, nurses' notes, patient teaching plans, utilization reviews, assessment data, and patient histories using computerized nursing information systems in required clinical courses (see Chapter Eleven). All of the above mentioned activities could be graded, evaluated for individual learning, evaluated for extra bonus points or assessed for satisfactory achievement measures.

The ethical/legal/moral oriented course offers great content for a traditional formal paper. There is a need for research papers in nursing curricula providing that these papers are meaningful to the understanding of course content and development of thinking and communication skills. Students could write a formal paper that addresses an ethical issue, presents an ethical position and argument, and a solution along with the prediction of the consequences of the solution. Formal papers should be graded.

Another writing-across-the-curriculum theme is writing for professional growth and research. This theme is important because it reflects the American Nurses Association Standards for Practice (1991) and the American Nurses Association Code for Nurses (1985). These dictate that nurses use research findings in practice, assume responsibility and accountability for individual nursing judgments and actions, consider factors related to safety, effectiveness, and cost in planning and delivering patient care, and collaborate with the patient, significant others, and healthcare providers in providing patient care. Junior or senior level courses that contain content related to adult health, community mental health, child nursing, maternal/infant nursing research, and leadership/management provide a realistic setting for writing-to-learn strategies aimed at enhancing professional growth and research. One highly successful strategy involves faculty mentoring students in preparing manuscripts for publication. Students utilize many writing-to-learn techniques, like brainstorming, dialectics, freewritings, and drafting while learning the process of writing for publication. This project also enhances communication skills and stimulates the faculty to engage in research and writing for publication (see Chapter Five). Bonus points are great for this project.

Written critiques of nursing research literature provide focused writing sessions for students while learning about the research process and current research topics in nursing practice and education. Students could present their critiques to nursing staff on units that pertain to clinical practice. This provides a professional audience and an opportunity for education and practice to communicate that could initiate new clinical research ideas (see Chapter Twelve). Critiques should be graded since research must be applicable to practice, realistic, and valid if it is to add to the knowledge base of the profession.

Individual or group writing projects work well in a community mental health course. A group writing-to-learn project that produces an asthma screening and prevention program or a health promotion program related to good mental health practices for implementation in a community school-based clinic utilizes many writing-to-learn techniques that assist students to learn more about community health needs for specific populations. This project should be graded and the individual or group should present their program(s) to the nurses at the clinic, the school board that governs the clinic, and to other students. This gives students an opportunity to write for different audiences and enhances realism in practice and communication skills and bridges a gap between education and practice.

Leadership/management courses provide students with the opportunity to write critical paths for practice and nursing care delivery models that address cost, collaborative care management, and patient care issues for hospitals.

When incorporating writing-to-learn across the curriculum, special attention needs to be given to possibilities for linkages for writing activities between clinical courses. For example, many papers written in those first courses could be rewritten in the more advanced courses, incorporating new knowledge and developing a more complex understanding of the subject matter (Allen, Bowers, & Diekelmann, 1989). A paper on complications of abdominal surgery could change if the patient were a child compared to an elder patient. Health promotion programs, skills procedures, critical paths, patient education plans, and needs assessment reports could be written for hospital-based and homebound patients.

Journal writing can be an extension of class notes, the focus on one topic or broadly on one's feelings. In lecture/discussion courses that require understanding the relationships between concepts, such as the concept of caring and actual application of nursing knowledge in clinical settings, journal writing has been found to be effective (Hahnemann, 1986).

The use of dialectics, brainstorming, microthemes, scenarios, and quickwrites are beneficial in across-the-curriculum writing-to-learn programs. Dialectics require the writer to record notes from readings on the left side of a page and comments or questions about the material read on the right side of a page. Nursing students can grasp more meaning from journal articles and research papers by using dialectics.

Brainstorming and scenarios are very helpful in teaching students application of the nursing process. For example, the instructor reads a hypothetical patient situation and asks small groups to generate written lists of observation cues that support development of problem lists that leads to a nursing diagnostic statement. This sparks sharing of ideas and critical thinking. In clinical courses, students could write lists of innovative nursing interventions for a given patient situation which in turn could generate new research ideas.

Quickwrites can serve as a check list for individual understanding of a lecture topic for any class. The writing-to-learn activities are endless.

Educators need to carefully examine writing at the curricular level. Undergraduate students need more practice in writing as they progress through the curriculum. Writing-to-learn across the curriculum can happen with or without additional funding. This innovative curriculum movement requires dedicated faculty who are truly interested in student learning to achieve high-quality outcomes in the development of critical thinking, communication, and research skills necessary for professional maturity.

Faculty need to own and operationalize their writing-across-the-curriculum program. Faculty must go beyond utilization of and participation in writing-to-learn curricular activities. Serious attention needs to be given to critical assessment of student outcomes. Do writing-to-learn strategies enhance learning (Walvoord, 1996)? Bowers and McCarthy (1993) found that writing-to-learn strategies appeared to enhance the evolution of cognitive skills in nursing students while, at the same time, these strategies brought student and teacher much closer together, invigorating both. Curricular changes related to writing that focused on problem solving and communication concepts in an engineering program of study led to a number of positive changes in faculty attitudes, according to a ten-year comparison of faculty attitudes about writing (Olds, 1990). Dobie and Poirrier, and Poirrier (1995) reported that students responded more positively to statements on their Writing to Learn Attitudinal Survey as a posttest after receiving writing-to-learn educational interventions than they did when the survey was administered as a pretest. Weber-Breaux and Poirrier (1994) reported that a writing strategy, family analysis improved student learning of family science concepts (see Chapter Fifteen). These are beginning research studies that test the effects of writing-to-learn and the whole WAC movement. Do faculty utilize writing-to-learn? Does writing-to-learn make a difference? How does writing-to-learn help students to learn? What are students learning as a result of writing-to-learn? Does writing-to-learn impact student/teacher relationships? How are faculty rewarded for using writing-to-learn? Students, faculty, funding agencies, and the general public are demanding qualitative and quantifiable answers.

REFERENCES

Allen, D. G., Bowers, B., & Diekelmann, N. (1989). Writing to learn: A reconceptualization of thinking and writing in the nursing curriculum. *Journal of Nursing Education, 28*(1), 6–11.

American Nurses Association (ANA). (1985). *Code for nurses with interpretive statements.* Washington, DC: Author.

American Nurses Association (ANA). (1991). *Standards of clinical nursing practice.* Washington, DC: Author.

Bowers, B., & McCarthy, D. (1993). Developing analytic thinking skills in early undergraduate education. *Journal of Nursing Education, 32*(3), 107–114.

Bruffee, K. (1978). The Brooklyn plan: Attaining intellectual growth through peer group tutoring. *Liberal Education, 64,* 447–468.

Dobie, A., & Poirrier, G. (1995). Evaluating writing-to-learn: Does it work?, In *Proceedings of the Second National Conference on Writing Across the Curriculum.* Charleston, SC: University of Charleston, Clemson University, The Citadel.

Hahnemann, B. (1986). Journal writing: A key to promoting critical thinking in nursing students. *Journal of Nursing Education, 25*(5), 213–215.

National League for Nursing. (1992). *Criteria and guidelines for the evaluation of baccalaureate and higher degree programs in nursing.* New York: Author. (Publication No. 15-2474)

Olds, B. M. (1990). Does a writing program make a difference? A ten-year comparison of faculty attitudes about writing. *Writing Program Administration, 14*(1–2), 27–40.

Poirrier, G. P. (1995). Interdisciplinary research: Evaluating writing to learn in the nursing curriculum. *Nursing Connections, 8*(3), 47–53.

Walvoord, B. E. (1996). The future of WAC. *College English, 58*(1), 58–79.

Weber-Breaux, J. G., & Poirrier, G. P. (1994). Family analysis: Effectiveness of a writing strategy in family science learning. *Family Science Review, 7*(3 & 4), 105–112.

Chapter Five

WRITING FOR PROFESSIONAL GROWTH

Melinda Granger Oberleitner, DNS, RN, OCN
Paula C. Broussard, RN, MN

WW riting-to-learn activities in nursing curricula are useful tools. In addition to facilitating learning and critical thinking, specific writing-to-learn activities in preprofessional curricula such as nursing can produce graduate nurses who are prepared to participate in professional communication at the beginning of their career. As students move through the preprofessional curriculum, they are able to make the transition from writing-to-learn to writing-to-communicate. This chapter will describe a specific writing-to-learn technique, writing for publication. Students are guided as they move from the level of personal interpretation, which is accomplished through assignments such as journal writing, to a higher level of objective analysis required in the publication process.

Writing for publication utilizes prose that is reader based and uses the formal language of the professional community (Young, 1993). It requires writing for a distant audience, encourages students to create and organize themes and ideas, and requires them to defend their ideas. Students are required to utilize the process of analytical thinking in developing a critical understanding of the professional base. The students must then develop the ability to communicate this knowledge to various professional audiences.

The theoretical foundation for this project was based on Perry's model of the stages of adult cognitive development, which provides a map for tracking students' thinking skills and the way they view knowledge (Perry, 1978). This WTL project was designed to foster contextualism, the process whereby students begin to understand that knowledge is contextual in nature. Writing encourages the student to think in abstraction, and to conceptualize, elaborate, substantiate, analyze, generalize, and interpret.

Methods

As an alternative to a clinical reasoning exam (2.5% of course grade), baccalaureate students enrolled in a senior nursing course were offered the opportunity to work with faculty mentors in preparing a manuscript for publication. Students were encouraged to recount clinical experiences in a format of their choosing (grand rounds, case studies, etc.). Students were expected to prepare a publishable manuscript adhering to a predetermined timetable with faculty assistance (Table 5.1). The project was originally funded by an intramural instructional grant.

The objectives of this project were to:

- Enhance learning via principles of writing-to-learn.
- Foster analytical thinking by students through use of the process of writing for publication.
- Reinforce prior learning through critical analysis of clinical experiences.
- Increase professional identity of nursing students through faculty mentoring.
- Emphasize the power of sharing "stories" as a valid method of professional communication.

Table 5.1
Sample Timetable for Completion

December	Solicit student and faculty volunteers for participation.
January	Faculty orientation to project.
January	Finalize faculty/student participation.
January	Publication workshop.
February	Student will have selected mentor and topic.
February	Format and target journal selected; query letter to target publication.
April	Final draft of manuscript complete.
April	Publish samples of student writings.

As the initial step in project implementation, faculty and students were oriented to the project and given general information on publication in a four-hour work shop. The project timetable was discussed, evaluation tools were disseminated (Table 5.2), and students were introduced to specific faculty research and publication interests. Students could then select mentors based on specific areas of faculty interest.

RESULTS/EVALUATION

Initially, twelve senior students volunteered to participate in the project. The students elected to work singly and in pairs. Eight faculty with varying clinical backgrounds were selected by students to serve as writing mentors. Faculty were selected on the basis of interest in the project and previous experience with the publication process.

All of the students adhered to the predetermined timetable for completion of the project. Students, working in conjunction with faculty, selected a topic for the manuscript and researched journals that would be suitable for publication of that topic. With editorial assistance from mentors, students composed and mailed query letters to editorial staff of selected journals. All of the participants identified themselves as students participating in a project under the direction of faculty mentors. Most of the journals queried responded to the students' letters.

During the time students were awaiting responses to query letters, the authors were encouraged to begin drafts of the manuscripts. Students met weekly or biweekly with their writing mentors to continually refine the articles. Once interest from journal editorial staff was determined, faculty assisted the students in targeting one journal for submission of the completed manuscript.

After selection of one target journal, the faculty assisted students in complying with specific guidelines for authors as stipulated by the journal. At this time, the focus was to modify the draft article to conform to suggested length, format, and style as recommended

Table 5.2
A Faculty Mentoring Writing-to-Learn Strategy Project Evaluation Tool

---

Student Name: _____

Faculty Name: _____

Point Total: _____

Professional Role   (40 Total Points)

(2.5 points)	1. Student actively participated in the WTL Publication Seminar.
(2.5 points)	2. Student initiated the selection of a faculty mentor.
(7.5 points)	3. Student initiated, collaborated, and negotiated with mentor to select topic area/focus.
(7.5 points)	4. Student initiated target journal selection(s).
(20 points)	5. Student initiated and actively participated in *all* phases of the writing project.

Implementation Phase   (40 Total Points)

(7.5 points)	1. Student initiated the composition of query letter; final draft to faculty for approval.
(7.5 points)	2. Student initiated and consulted with mentor on a weekly basis (or as determined by faculty) with drafts and revisions of the manuscripts.
(25 points)	3. Manuscript submitted in publishable form to mentor by deadline date.

    a. Manuscript submitted in formal format, i.e., using computer, printer output, tables.

    b. Accurate, current, and pertinent references utilized.

    c. Appropriate format/publication style for target journal utilized (Example: APA format).

    d. Organization, clarity, completeness of ideas, correct grammar, spelling, and punctuation.

    e. Contribution to the nursing literature; scholarliness.

Evaluation Phase   (20 Total Points)

(20 points)	1. Student submitted a formal written self-evaluation of their role in the project to faculty mentor and project coordinators by deadline date.

by the guidelines for authors. Once those refinements were completed, seven articles developed by the senior students were formally submitted to national journals for publication.

While awaiting responses to the submissions, students and faculty mentors completed formal evaluations of the writing project. Faculty were responsible for conducting formative evaluations during the entire process. Mentors were also asked to complete an evaluation tool based on the project objectives. Finally, faculty were to assign a student grade for the project utilizing the evaluation tool designed by project coordinators.

As part of the formal project evaluation process, students completed a tool designed by the project coordinators to evaluate satisfaction with the learning process. All students and faculty participating in the project evaluated the experience as a resounding success. For example, neither faculty nor students felt that the project was too time consuming. All participants agreed that critical thinking and analytical thinking could be enhanced using principles of writing-to-learn.

Two other activities were conducted while awaiting responses from editorial staffs. A compendium of the students' writings was printed and distributed to all junior and senior nursing students in the college of nursing. The compendia were also distributed to the university's vice president for academic affairs and to all members of the university's Writing-Across-the-Curriculum (WAC) committee. This compendium, which featured student articles accompanied by their photographs, was funded by grant monies received by the project coordinators.

As a means of showcasing the success of the project, a "Meet the Authors" reception was organized. All College of Nursing faculty, students, and staff were invited as well as many university officials. Student writings were exhibited at this event and students were given the opportunity to verbally relate their experiences with the project. The event was well attended.

Toward the end of that spring semester and through the summer months, students began to receive responses to the submissions. Of the seven articles submitted for publication, five (71%) were accepted for publication. Articles were selected for publication in journals, such as *Nursing, Minority Nurse, Pediatric Nurse, Caring,* and *Imprint.* Both student authors and faculty mentors were overwhelmed by the high publication acceptance rate.

As a result of the success of the initial project and increased interest and excitement on the part of other students and faculty, the project was extended for subsequent semesters. Several faculty members expressed disappointment to project coordinators that they were not selected as writing mentors by students.

The success of the project continues to generate excitement in the university and nursing communities. An article describing the project was published in *Scribe,* the Writing Across the Curriculum university-wide publication. Other articles about the project have been published in print media including the university's student newspaper, local newspapers, and newspapers in each student's hometown. Some of the students have been asked by nursing leaders in the community to share their writing experiences with their staff.

The senior students who were participants in the initial project have now graduated. All expressed that they felt a distinct competitive advantage in competing for a position in a depressed job market because of their participation in the project. All included a citation of their publication in their resumes and portfolios.

CONCLUSION

This project ignited tremendous interest in the writing-to-learn process. It led to increased publications among College of Nursing faculty. The project was an unqualified success and a commitment was made to make the experience available for prospective authors in succeeding classes.

The ultimate significance of this project is the development of professional nurses who are prepared to participate in the publication process. In any profession, writing for publication is of paramount importance for the development of the profession in general and for its individual members. Simply put, "the future of the nursing profession depends on writing" (Styles, 1981).

REFERENCES

Perry, W. (1978). Growth in the making of meaning: Youth into adulthood. In A. Chickaring (Ed.), *The future of American colleges.* San Francisco: Jossey-Bass.

Styles, M. M. (1981). Why publish. *Image: The Journal of Nursing Scholarship, 10,* 28–32.

Young, A. (1993, March 19). *Writing across the curriculum.* Paper presented at the University of Southwestern Louisiana, Lafayette, LA.

Chapter Six

WRITING-TO-LEARN COMMUNICATION

Zoe New, MSN, RN, CETN, CRRN

*C*ommunication is one of the most important and rewarding aspects of nursing. Through communication, nurses are able to experience an intimacy with clients and colleagues, which few professionals experience. Through focusing on the client's needs and feelings, nurses are able to help them heal, participate in their care, solve their own problems, clarify their thoughts and needs, and move toward their human potential. Communication is an area where nurses can experience autonomy, really connect with other human beings, and truly make a difference in people's lives.

One can hardly imagine how nursing as a helping profession centered on the client's needs could even exist without communication. Nurses use communication as a vehicle for exchanging information, thoughts, and feelings, and as a means of influencing behaviors. Kozier, Erb, and Olivieri's (1991) text, *Fundamentals of Nursing*, describes communication as "essential for the establishment of the nurse-client relationship" and "a significant aspect of nursing practice" (p. 247).

Everything nurses do involves communication. Whether they are assessing clients or situations, planning, carrying out, or evaluating care, they must quickly establish a nurse-client relationship. To do this, they must communicate effectively and establish a sense of trust and partnership. This is very complex and difficult because clients come from diverse socioeconomic backgrounds, settings, and have multiple, unmet needs. These clients and their families are expected to assume an active and informed role in the prevention, maintenance, and recovery aspects of their care. Nurses must establish what the PEW Health Professions Commission (1991) calls "relationship-centered care" where information, feelings, and concerns are exchanged and the nurse and client share an understanding of the meaning of illness. These "relationship skills" enable nurses to be vehicles for health and healing.

According to Arnold and Boggs (1995) communication is "the matrix of the nurse-client relationship" (p. 19). Virtually all nursing theorists agree that effective communication skills are necessary to carry out the successful practice of nursing. Several theorists' conceptual frameworks even focus on interpersonal relationships. Nurses are legally and professionally bound by virtue of the nurse-client relationship and their state Nurse Practice Acts to provide a reasonable standard of nursing care using the nursing process. In order to carry out each step of the nursing process, nurses must communicate effectively. The National League of Nursing considers communication so important that they have identified communication as one of the three required outcome criteria that baccalaureate nursing programs must address for accreditation.

All of us communicate in some form or another every day. If asked, most of us would say we know how to communicate and nursing students are no exception. The second semester junior level nursing students who are in my communication class have written papers in English and composition courses and given speeches in speech classes. They are sure they already know how to communicate. However, as they progress in the course, many find they are not the communication experts they thought they were. Several students have said that they thought the course was for "other" students who did not already know how to communicate. They felt that they were needlessly taking a required course because of "other" students' deficiencies. They also felt the communication course was a waste of time they could have spent practicing the "hands-on skills" really needed by nurses. When the students complete the course, they are aware of the importance of communication skills in their nursing practice, and can use basic communication strategies. Most become aware of how difficult effective communication really is. They also learn that the only way they know that they have correctly perceived someone's message is to check their perception with the communicator. To make this transition requires that the students observe themselves, reflect upon their behavior, and change certain behavior and beliefs. Not only do they have to learn new communication knowledge and skills, but they have to apply them in their nursing practice and unlearn old, comfortable communication skills.

When I was first asked to teach a core course focusing on therapeutic communication and became aware of the objectives, I began to explore teaching strategies that utilized principles of adult learning. The traditional lecture, writing pages of nurse-client dialogue, and an informational term paper did not seem to be effective teaching strategies to accomplish the course objectives. All but one of the objectives included application to practice. The students were to be able to apply communication processes, conflict resolution, and critical thinking skills in personal and nursing situations. To me, this meant that all sixty students should be able to actually practice and perform the communication skills they were going to learn. I have used writing-to-learn strategies along with the experiential teaching-learning process suggested by Arnold and Boggs (1995) to accomplish this. Writing integrates very nicely with experiential learning and augments the discussion and reflection exercises contained in the text. The writing activities that I will describe are for the purpose of helping the student think, learn about themselves, and learn to communicate rather than writing to communicate information.

The first writing activity is a modification of process recording. The process recording contains only therapeutic responses rather than a narrative and is combined with classroom role playing. Students read and view an interactive video on therapeutic communication and communication facilitators and barriers. They then write three examples of facilitating responses they made to a client, classmate, or nurse during their clinical practice the following week. During the actual clinical experience, the students have so much going on that they find it difficult to do more than jot down a short interaction. Initially, few students are capable of sustaining a therapeutic interaction for very long. They focus on their own performance and psychomotor skills. It is not until later that they can focus on what the client really said and meant. The three interactions are to be no longer than the one-page form in their syllabus. The form has columns for client's remarks, student's remarks, student's perception of the client, and analysis. The analysis includes the nurse's thoughts and feelings about the interaction, recurrent themes, and whether or not the response was therapeutic. If the response was not therapeutic, the student is to write a therapeutic response. Each column has specific instructions to guide the students' writing and analysis. During the next class period, the students discuss their interactions and submit them to the instructor. The students complete the exercise twice before and once after the midterm exam.

The students share their first process recording with a classmate seated nearby for feedback. If the response was not therapeutic, the two of them write a revised response that is therapeutic or improved. The students then form groups of six to eight persons to share their interactions and pick the best one. The best interaction is then role played for the whole class. Discussion and suggestions follow each interaction. Sometimes I participate in the role playing and model therapeutic responses. The revisions and the classmate's name are on the process recording and submitted to the instructor for feedback and a grade. I make no effort to prevent the students from making revisions during the role playing and discussion. The students receive written feedback and a grade when the instructor returns the papers the following week. The grade is the average of the grades of the two individuals who worked together on the process recording. Each process recording constitutes 3% of the student's total grade. I would like to have these writing exercises ungraded but have found that the students take graded assignments more seriously. I would also like to eliminate grading these myself and rely instead on the students' grading and providing feedback to one another. Unfortunately, I found that the students are not assertive or knowledgeable enough to give each other the depth of feedback they need when the assignments are due. I plan to continue working on this by making the criteria more explicit and helping the students learn the criteria. The students address assertiveness as a communication process later in the semester.

The second and third process recording include the same elements as the first two, plus the students must now determine the level of empathy. They also try to reach level four or five on Carkhuff's empathy scale (as cited in Arnold & Boggs, 1995). The same process of sharing their written interactions and revisions with a classmate; then meeting in groups and choosing the best example of empathetic interaction occurs. The best from each group is again role played for the entire class for demonstration, discussion, suggestion, and revision. These interactions are much more difficult and interesting because the students must elicit the client's feelings. This is very difficult for many students because they focus on their own feelings, level of comfort, and responses. Many students are very uncomfortable with the whole subject and presence of feelings. Writing helps them begin to make sense of their emotions and thoughts in a way many have never experienced. The student is able to look at the interaction closely and from a distance. This allows the student to view the situation from the perspectives of the client, classmate, and instructor as well as their own. From here students can explore the meaning of the situation and actually grasp the meaning of empathy with personal and meaningful insights.

According to Berthoff (1982), the act of composition itself helps writers make sense of what they are trying to write. Bandman and Bandman (1995) also note the value of putting language into writing so nurses can think critically about what they are writing by examining it and reflecting on the meaning and hidden feelings. I have found, as did Emig (1977), that writing "represents a unique mode of learning—not merely valuable, not merely special, but unique." (p. 122). It is unique because writing makes our thoughts visible and concrete so that we are able to manipulate, modify, and interact with them. According to Fulwiler (1987) writing is the only way most of us can develop and extend our thoughts because this is the only way we can attend to multiple thoughts at one time. If we do not write out our communication, we lose much of what is said. I have found this visibility necessary for the students to be able to believe as well as assess and analyze their interactions. From here they can reflect upon their communication, and evaluate and revise their responses. They can experiment with alternatives and compose responses that will be useful when they find themselves in similar situations.

Both the student and the instructor are able to follow the student's progress by comparing and contrasting the process recording with earlier and later writings. We are able to explore together any learning gaps and areas needing improvement. The students are able to receive individual attention and honest, empathetic, and respectful feedback that would not otherwise be possible in large classes. Grading the papers proceeds very quickly because the papers are short. I have found that the sharing of writing between student and teacher helps to establish a relationship that enhances students learning therapeutic communication. My observations are supported by the findings of Karns and Schwab (1982). The students surveyed in their study listed empathy, congruent messages, and respect along with availability and teaching ability as behaviors that promoted a positive relationship with their teacher.

Students need to be able to see the communication errors and successes repeatedly and in different contexts before they can write therapeutic responses to exam questions or use them in their clinical practice. This is particularly true in the areas where students must replace their usual responses with newly learned therapeutic responses. Behaviors that students frequently have difficulty eliminating are unwarranted reassurance offerings, advice giving, problem solving for others, and playing detective. Many times students try to elicit information so they can give advice or solve the person's problem. Students find it particularly difficult to switch from problem solving for clients to helping clients solve their own problems.

To evaluate students' learning, there are six questions on the midterm examination asking the students to write their response to situations or statements similar to those practiced in class. The exam is worth 20% of the course grade. The remainder of the exam consists of multiple choice questions asking students to pick the best response. This is a sample question.

A 30-year-old male with a spouse and two children comes into the hospital for possible liver failure. He says to you, "Having this yellow jaundice is the last straw. You live a good clean life, eat right, don't smoke or drink and look where it gets you." Write your best response reflecting the content and feeling of what the client has said.

Another tool to foster communication skills involves writing a one-page paper describing how students can apply the information on "self-talk" from a nursing journal. I chose an article for the students to respond to which contained information concerning feelings since this is a difficult area for many students. Students needed to be aware of their "self-talk" to help them reduce their stress so they can focus more on their communication skills and strategies. I also hoped to help debunk cognitive distortions that cause them and their clients grief. In order to have something to write, the student must reflect on the meaning of the article and how it related to them and their nursing practice. This enables the student to personalize the content and assimilate it into their lives and practice. Writing forces students, even quiet students, to take a position on issues, present themselves to others, and learn that it is not a catastrophe if others do not agree with them. Usually students are proud of their work and abilities and optimistically await the return of their papers. The students' high scores on this paper affirm their suspicion that they did better than they thought they could. The score counts for 3% of their course grade.

The final writing-to-learn strategy involves the students forming groups to make a video in which they role play a conflict resolution. The students write a paper analyzing the roles of group members' decision making as they plan and make the video. They read the content on the subject in their text and syllabus before coming to class. During class, the students form groups of three to four persons to outline the content for their video. While half of the groups plan their video, the other half of the groups observe and practice analyzing the group roles and decision making. The groups switch activities with one another after 30 minutes so each group has an opportunity to participate in both activities. The students' syllabus contains a content outline, a guide for their analysis, and some summary materials on groups that the students find helpful. During the group activities, the instructor should move from group to group to ask and answer questions. Individual students take notes on the group process as the groups meet outside of class to continue working on their videos. The directions in the syllabus specify that the student's analysis must include a clear description of the group process, application of the analysis to nursing practice, and the student's conclusions. All of these areas are described in detail. The students comment on their discoveries about themselves and fellow classmates as well as the group process. The roles, leadership, conflict resolution, and decision-making styles that emerge surprise them. Completing this project affirms the students' belief in their ability to complete a project and work both independently and cooperatively. The students work hard on this paper and video and their grades reflect their work. Each of these projects is worth 20% of their course grade.

I have experienced the positive benefits of writing to learn as I have struggled to write and think about it while writing this chapter.

REFERENCES

Arnold, E., & Boggs, K. U. (1995). *Interpersonal skills: Professional communication for nurses* (2nd ed.). Philadelphia, PA: W. B. Saunders.

Bandman, E. L., & Bandman, B. (1995). *Critical thinking in nursing* (2nd ed.). Norwalk, CT: Appleton & Lange.

Berthoff, A. E. (1982). *Forming, thinking, and writing: The composing imagination.* Upper Montclair, NJ: Boynton/Cook.

Emig, J. (1977). Writing as a mode of learning. *College Composition for Nurses, 28,* 122–128.

Fulwiler, T. (1987). *Teaching with writing.* Portsmouth, NH: Boynton/Cook.

Karns, P. S., & Schwab, T. A. (1982). Therapeutic communication and clinical instruction. *Nursing Outlook, 30,* 39–43.

Kozier, B., Erb, G., & Olivieri, R. (1991). *Fundamentals of nursing: Concepts, process and practice.* (4th ed.). New York: Addison-Wesley.

PEW Health Professions Commission. (1991). *Health America: Practitioner for 2005.* Durham, NC: Duke University Medical Center.

Chapter Seven

JOURNAL WRITING IN NURSING

Susan W. Reynolds, RN, MS

*A*n important criterion set forth by the National League for Nursing as one standard for measuring the quality of an educational program is the critical thinking skills of its graduates. Unfortunately, research in education indicates that critical thinking does not "just happen" to students (Beyer, 1987). Activities such as reading, discussing, and writing about subject matter provide the student opportunities for thinking, but these approaches often do not lead to the development of critical thinking skills. Beyer (1987) proposes that educators need to teach thinking by engaging the students in activities that require the kinds of thinking we want them to develop.

Writing-to-learn across the curriculum programs emphasize the importance of using writing to enhance communication and critical thinking skills of the students. In clinical practicums at all levels of nursing education, writing in clinical journals is a common assignment. The clinical journal is a written record of the student nurse that reflects attitudes, feelings, and expansion of his or her cognitive learning that occurs throughout the particular nursing course (Callister, 1993). Fulwiler (1987) proposes that journals are neither a diary or a class notebook; rather they are both an objective and subjective chronicle. The clinical journal can thus become a valuable opportunity for educators to teach thinking directly by involving students actively in analyzing and evaluating their clinical experiences (Brown & Sorrell, 1993).

Students in an undergraduate baccalaureate nursing program at the University of Southwestern Louisiana are asked to keep clinical journals throughout their program of study. Entries include but are not limited to their personal learning objectives for the day, descriptive observations of their particular situation, their feelings and emotions of their varied experiences, ethical concerns, and particular challenges they experienced. Consent to reproduce various journal entries was given by the students for use in this chapter.

Many faculty report that students' journals are often disappointing in that they do not reflect the anticipated critical thinking that is so desired (Brown & Sorrell, 1993). Conversely, some students complain about the requirement that they write and submit weekly journals to their instructors. Other students begin by writing enthusiastically in their journals, but after several weeks, they seem to become "burned out" with the activity. Other students regard journal writing as "busy work" and not worthy of the same attention of other academic papers. Procrastinating about journal writing is another problem and can result in sketchy and omitted entries. Finally, some students do not understand what is expected of them in their journal writing, and often these individuals produce mere recordings of their clinical day.

This chapter will focus on ways to enhance the experience of nursing students in maintaining clinical journals and on ways to help prevent or minimize the common problems associated with journal writing. Information contained in this chapter is based on research in nursing and education, as well as my own experience as a clinical instructor. Journal excerpts contained in this chapter were provided by junior and senior level baccalaureate nursing students.

First, faculty need to identify for students the purpose and expectations for the journal assignments, and communicate this information clearly to the student. The clinical journal provides students a guided opportunity to "think aloud" on paper, reflecting on their own perceptions or analysis of the situations they encounter in the clinical area. As a result, they learn to synthesize theory and practice, apply relevant research and literature to clinical situations, and raise questions and concerns for further study (Brown & Sorrell, 1993). Clinical journals should not be viewed as formal, scholarly papers, but as on-going dialogues between students and faculty. As a result, typical academic concerns such as grammar, spelling, and sentence construction are not particularly relevant. Typical guidelines that I give to students are as follows:

> Your clinical journal is an important communication tool. It is a personal, student-centered recording of significant aspects of

your clinical day. The journal provides an opportunity to share with your clinical instructor theory and research obtained in the classroom that you were able to apply in the clinical area. Entries should be made for each clinical day and should be written as soon as possible following the clinical experience. Date each entry and keep them chronologically in a notebook or looseleaf. Be sure the entries are legible.

Suggestions as to what the students may include in their entries are as follows:

1. One or more objectives or goals for the day. (These may be personal goals or objectives related to those identified in the course syllabus.)
2. Significant activities that occurred during the course of the clinical day.
3. Personal reactions to the clinical experience. Include your thoughts and feelings.
4. Ethical concerns that may have arisen during the course of your activities.
5. Meaningful interactions or experiences that you may have had with other healthcare providers, positive or negative.

From the above guidelines, several benefits of the clinical journal to the student become apparent. The journal provides the student with the opportunity to explore significant aspects of the clinical experience that are meaningful to them. It focuses on the unique experiences of the student nurse as a method of learning in a self-actualizing framework (Callister, 1993).

The journal provides the student an opportunity to release emotions and feelings about clinical experiences in a nonthreatening manner as illustrated by these entries:

One thing I have learned from this client is to never judge someone solely from what the other nurses tell you about them. The nursing staff thought that this client could not speak or understand English very well, they stated that she was illiterate and was a "difficult patient." None of this was true. All this client needed was to be treated like a human being. She wanted information about her condition and reassurance. I noticed at least three staff members, including both nurses and aides, who came into the room, spoke to her, and yet never once made eye contact with her.

Or as another student reveals:

On our arrival at the nursery, a black male infant was under a warmer. When I spotted him, I noted his arms were extended at his sides and his legs were extended away from his body. I felt a panic rush through me as I knew his position was not normal. I really was afraid I was looking at a dead baby. I looked for signs of life and noted his abdomen moving so I knew he was alive. He had been born an hour earlier, but had severe acrocyanosis, nasal flaring, flaccidity of his extremities, cyanotic coloration of his face, and was hard to stimulate. I couldn't help but worry about this baby the whole time we were at the hospital and he has been on my mind since then. I wonder if he improved or got worse. This experience makes me wonder how I will react if this or any other baby that I care for dies. It really scares me.

Identifying what is right or good in a situation promotes ethical understanding. In their clinical journals, nursing students can apply the principles of ethical decision making that they learned in the classroom to clinical situations that pose ethical dilemmas. The students are encouraged to explore new ways of thinking and responding in clinical practice. For example, one student writes:

I think this particular patient I cared for was getting very poor care from the nursing staff. She sat in her own feces for 2 to 3 hours because her nurse didn't come when she first called, and the client did not want to bother her again. Even in her routine daily care, the nursing aides would not wash her hair the day before I took care of her, they just said no! I would be so frustrated in her situation, everyone else decided what was best for her, regardless of her feelings.

The clinical instructor responded to this student to be careful not to get too involved in the client's criticisms until more information and specific questions could be asked. Then the student could reflect on the situation and a plan of action could be instituted.

Journal writing helps to foster the reflective skills of students. Reflection can be viewed as a deliberate and conscious activity that permits the individual to contemplate behavior and events and responses to them. Schon (1984) proposes that the contemplation of past or current behavior and experiences facilitates future action. As one student reflects:

> If you really *listen* to this client, and talk to her, not at her, you will find that she is confused. She is not sleeping well, she is taking tranquilizers, and so she does forget and needs reminding and reinforcement. I don't know too much about the availability of support groups, but this client and her husband really need to talk to someone who has been through this situation before, to tell them what to expect, to show them that life can go on normally; to basically give them hope. [The client had suffered a major stroke.] I had a long talk with her son, he just did not want to believe she would never walk again. We talked about things that his mother would be able to do, we discussed wheelchair ramps, hand-controlled cars, and other assistive devices. We both felt that his mother would do better in the hospital if she had the same staff members assigned to her as frequently as possible. She was very agitated with all the different people caring for her, she needed more continuity and familiarity.

Or as another student reflects:

> This was a wonderful experience for me. Mrs. K. came to the United States after working in a labor camp during the Holocaust. She wonders, "Why do I live so long only to get this monster inside of me? Why must I suffer so? Why can I not die quickly." Mrs. K. has outlived her husband and almost all of her friends. She does have two children; a daughter who lives in Houston and visits every other week or so, and a son who lives in Arkansas who is "uncomfortable with illness," so he never comes to visit. She is

so lonely. She was overjoyed to have a student nurse care for her this week. She shared many feelings with me. She alternated between funny, joyful replies to my questions to suddenly becoming fearful. I asked her what her greatest fear was and she replied that she did not want to suffer. I talked to her at length about the availability of medications to help make her more comfortable, and although at first she seemed doubtful, she later did call her nurse and ask for one of her PRN medications. Later after she was discharged from the hospital, I was allowed to make a home visit to Mrs. K. with the home health nurse assigned to her care. When we arrived, during the course of the conversation, Mrs. K. wanted to know if the aide could help her clean up her kitchen. She was very concerned about it. Carroll, the home health nurse told her that it wasn't the aide's job, but she could ask her. Mrs. K. replied, "All of my life, I am strong. I help others. It is a strange thing to rely on the kindness of others now." We left her house but I just could not get her off my mind. I then asked another student if she would go back to the house with me when we were done with clinical for the day so we could help Mrs. K. clean her kitchen. Carroll, the home health nurse overheard my conversation, thought a minute, and said, "Let's all go." When we got back to Mrs. K.'s and told her our reason for returning, she began to laugh and cry. Her face was such a vision of joy, she said, "My heart is melting from your kindness, you are such wonderful girls." She later stated, "I wonder why God let me live so long?" I replied, "Maybe so that you could touch my life." She looked at me, took my hands in hers and said, "Then God has blessed us both."

I am not the kind of person who cries very easily, but tears come to my eyes again as I write this. Sometimes I feel so rich. This was one of those passing moments in life that make you feel happier, stronger, and see life more clearly than ever before.

Students will vary in their ability to be reflective in their clinical journals. Their skill may be influenced by cultural and gender factors, as well as the availability of reflective role models. It is for this reason that I will on occasion ask a particularly reflective student to share a particular part of their clinical journal with their peers.

Particular interests of the students will affect their motivation to reflect. Few clinical students are equally interested in all of their clinical areas and experiences. As a consequence, one should not expect all journal entries to be of equal length and quality. In addition, all students are not proficient in reflective writing; however, reflective skills can be improved if students are encouraged and given opportunities to test and question their beliefs about clinical practice (Hahnemann, 1986).

A major factor influencing this development of reflective skill in the student is the level of trust between the student and clinical instructor. If students are not allowed to express their ideas freely without risk of negative consequences, they will write to impress or please the instructor, not to learn from the reflective experience. Where there exists an environment of mutual respect and trust, clinical journals provide the students with an opportunity to test their ideas, to inquire, and to discover their own voices. Writing in an open honest manner, however, can place the student in an extremely vulnerable position. Cameron and Mitchell (1993) report that a common fear of students is that they will write something that will alienate their instructor, the same individual on whom they rely for support and guidance in the clinical area. Students who know and trust their instructor to be nonjudgmental about their ideas and opinions will be more likely to risk self-disclosure in their journal entries. Students who are new to a clinical instructor may wait for positive evidence that the individual is truly nonjudgmental before they openly reflect in their journal entries.

Assigning a specific grade to the students' journal entries can provide another serious block to the reflective skill we hope to see in the clinical journals. In our current curriculum, no specific grade is assigned to the students' clinical journal, but it is a requirement that must be fulfilled if the student is to pass the clinical component of the course.

Although no specific grade is given for the clinical journals, provision of appropriate feedback to the students is necessary. It is not necessary to spend a great deal of time making spelling and grammatical corrections. Focusing too closely on grammatical aspects of the writing discourages students from trying out new ideas on paper. Faculty should instead provide one or two overall comments about the journal entry, encouraging the student to raise further questions to explore, and to analyze and evaluate their observations, and perceptions in relation to research and theory obtained from in and outside the classroom (Brown & Sorrell, 1993).

Clinical journals can also provide benefits for the faculty member. They help to provide insight into the personality and needs of the student nurse, and help to humanize the student-faculty relationship (Callister, 1993). The faculty member is assisted in the evaluation of progression in student learning in the areas of reflection and critical thinking as outlined previously. Progressive student growth can be seen in journal writings, evidence that learning has occurred.

Although the clinical journal may be seen as a time-consuming activity by both faculty and students at some point, the benefits and positive impact on student learning seem to outweigh any negative aspects of the activity. An informal survey was made of our current May 1996 graduates concerning their use of the clinical journals and some of their comments follow:

> The journals provided me an outlet for thoughts on the clinical experience that might not have been brought to my conscious arena had I not taken the time for the entry. I had some instructors that made very helpful comments in the journal, telling me my strengths, weaknesses, and encouraging me.

> I thought the journals were very beneficial to me. Even though they added to my work load, they allowed me to voice my feelings and experiences about important aspects of my clinical day. It also allowed the instructor to become aware of what was happening with me that day in clinical. I enjoyed the freedom of being able to choose important aspects of the day to write about rather than being told specifically what to write about.

> I think the journal writing activity was a very beneficial one for me because it allowed me to reflect on my clinical experiences of the day. I found them especially helpful when I was allowed to

write on what I considered meaningful to me. I did not find them as useful when the instructor dictated what was to be written, as I did not always feel the freedom then to express my true feelings.

CONCLUSION

In order to function effectively in today's changing healthcare environment, graduate nurses now need to be able to function as effective care-givers, client advocates, teachers, change agents, and leaders. The ability to reflect and think critically is of paramount importance to these individuals. It has been widely reported in the nursing literature that the use of student journals can be one very effective tool in helping to assist students to reflect and think critically about their learning experiences in the clinical area. Although maintaining a clinical journal requires a commitment from both student and faculty member, the benefits outweigh the necessary work commitment involved.

REFERENCES

Beyer, B. K. (1987). *Practical strategies for the teaching of thinking.* Lexington, MA: Allyn & Bacon.

Brown, H. N., & Sorrell, J. M. (1993). Use of clinical journals to enhance critical thinking. *Nurse Educator, 18*(5), 16–19.

Callister, L. C. (1993). The use of student journals in nursing education: Making meaning out of clinical experience. *Journal of Nursing Education, 32*(4), 185–186.

Cameron, B. L., & Mitchell, A. M. (1993). Reflective peer journals: Developing authentic nurses. *Journal of Advanced Nursing,* (18), 290–297.

Fulwiler, T. (1987). *Teaching with writing.* Upper Montclair, NJ: Boynton/Cook.

Hahnemann, B. K. (1986). Journal writing: A key to promoting critical thinking in nursing students. *Journal of Nursing Education,* (25), 213–215.

Schon, D. A. (1984). *The reflective practitioner.* New York: Basic Books.

Chapter Eight

PARTICIPATING IN LEARNING IN NURSING

Ann B. Dobie, EdD

Writing and nursing have never been strangers. Proficiency in keeping accurate records and making clear transactions has always been expected of the effective healthcare giver. Recent (and ongoing) changes in the field suggest that writing is likely to play an even larger role in nurses' professional lives in the coming decades. As healthcare broadens the scope of its services, moves to a more collaborative manner of operating, and shifts the responsibility for analysis of data, the ability to communicate effectively and to think critically about complex issues becomes increasingly important. The situation has already led most nurse educators to reconsider the curricula, teaching methods, and evaluation of their programs. For many of them, it has changed both the philosophies and practices that govern the preparation nurses are given for their careers.

In the past, most nursing programs used what Susan McLeod (1987) calls a "rhetorical approach" to writing (p. 20). That is, instructors asked students to produce papers, usually at the upper-division level, that conformed to the publishing conventions of the discipline. Because requiring students to write like nurses introduces them to forms of social behavior common to the occupation they will soon enter, the rhetorical approach remains a standard assignment in many classes. It helps them create a community of learners and writers not unlike the knowledge community in the discipline itself. They thereby become comfortable members of their professional discourse community.

Recently, however, writing in nursing classes has taken a new direction. McLeod calls it a "cognitive approach," as it "assumes that writing is a mode of thinking and learning," the way we "build our own knowledge structures . . . changing them as we receive new information" (p. 20). Learners are expected to be actively engaged in constructing what they know, not passive receivers and repeaters of what the instructor or the textbook knows. Where students have traditionally been asked to master a body of information, the cognitive approach asks them to replace memorization with thinking by practicing a variety of skills that they will need as nursing professionals: skills of analysis and synthesis, problem solving, and ethical choice. Finally, as the natural next step in the process, students are asked to make connections and discoveries, to take an inquiry stance that turns practitioners into researchers. Through written language, they carry thinking through its most complex processes, not simply rehearsing old knowledge, but reaching toward the new.

This chapter will tell the story of one course in which strategies to make students active co-participants in their learning fostered personal involvement in the subject matter, improved data comprehension, and encouraged critical thinking. In the end, their altered perspectives helped them more effectively grasp, integrate, construct, and articulate knowledge.

Charged with introducing nursing to beginning students, many of whom had chosen their major because they had heard there were jobs available in healthcare, the instructor faced a mission almost impossible. It was her job, over the course of the semester, to acquaint them with the characteristics of the nurse, describe past and expanding roles, explain current healthcare trends, and define professional involvement. In all these areas, she wanted to present nursing as a humanistic, caring discipline focused on human beings and their health. One semester she chose not simply to present the information, but to help her students discover it by using in-class writing activities that asked them to be reflective and inquiring participants in making knowledge. With the help of the director of writing at her university, she designed a course that would make class time more effective by including student activities that complemented the lectures and outside reading. Though she has varied her plans since that term, she has not returned to her earlier lecture and test techniques. She doesn't ever plan to.

She began with the first meeting of the semester. The room was long and narrow, the desks for seventy students arranged in straight lines emanating from the teacher's lecture podium but gradually becoming a disordered jumble at the back. The arrangement sent a clear message that truth and wisdom in Nursing 114 (Introduction to Basic Concepts) came from the front of the room.

The attentive students on the first row and the slouched ones in the back suggested that communication lost its vibrancy as it moved down the long, narrow corridors between the desks.

Hoping to energize the less than vigorous ambience, she invited students to focus on the purpose of the course. She led them to question their own roles in what they would be doing and to accept responsibility for what they would learn. To help them get started, she asked the class to write short answers to four questions:

1. Why do you want to be a nurse?
2. Name three personal goals you want to achieve in this course.
3. Do you think that writing is essential to success?
4. Explain why you like or don't like to write.

The classroom might not have encouraged student ownership of learning and knowledge, but the instructor's questions made it clear that personal investment in thinking about the important issues was expected.

As the semester developed, the instructor used other techniques to draw students into the work of making knowledge. She began classes with "admit slips," ten-minute nonstop writings that helped students to focus their thinking on the assigned reading for the day or on an upcoming discussion (Gere, 1985, p. 222). At the end of a period, she sometimes called for "exit slips" that summarized a class, allowing her to measure students' understanding of course material. On occasion she would interrupt a class to ask for a focused writing on some issue pertinent to the discussion, for example, the meaning of health or how nurses demonstrate ethical codes of behavior. Students wrote microthemes on 5 × 8-inch cards that pushed them to evaluate reading material and select the most important points in an assignment. They composed unsent letters to someone under study or as a person involved in the material being discussed. For example, they wrote letters to the creator of a character who is a nurse in a movie, book, or television show suggesting ways in which this character could more accurately represent a professional nurse. Sharing them with each other later, the students became more aware of public images of nurses, consumer healthcare expectations, and the powerful impact of public communication on current and future nursing practice in our society.

The strategies were never whimsically introduced. Each was planned and implemented following well-known principles of learning theory. For instance, recognizing that getting information in and out of long-term memory requires active work, the instructor designed the writing assignments to be multisensory and interactive—not passive exercises—and, whenever possible, to involve collaborative efforts. To make the material seem more alive, she framed the exercises so that students would recognize personal connections. Connections with other disciplines were also encouraged, bringing knowledge from other fields to bear on nursing. Finally, she moved sequentially from simple responses to increasingly complex ones that called for more difficult intellectual tasks.

Because writing assignments are effective only when they are introduced at the right time for the appropriate purpose, the instructor tied each one to course objectives, making certain that it underscored what was being taught at that point of the semester. Unless it served a meaningful purpose, it was dropped. She gave explanations of what the specific assignment was to explore, and sometimes suggested a systematic approach, lest the personal connections take students in directions not germane to the course work. The various assignments gave students opportunities to write for different (but specified) audiences and to try different genres.

Finally, the criteria for evaluation were clearly stated at the outset. Because the assignments were not to be graded in a traditional way (by heavy marking and correcting), it was important to define early on how students' work would be treated. Credit was earned for completion of assignments, but the emphasis was clearly placed on developing a teacher-student dialogue. Recognizing the importance of making timely responses, the instructor answered each student's work within a week, making positive suggestions that reinforced the relationship between the student's performance and the lesson's objective.

From the outset, the instructor sensed that something good was happening in the class. A greater vitality seemed to permeate the classroom as the long, straight rows of desks were broken up to facilitate sharing and collaboration. The greater degree of involvement could easily have been mistaken for disorder. The noise level in the classroom rose, and chairs sometimes had to be moved to accommodate new classroom arrangements. Passivity always looks more organized than activity, but the body language of the students was reassuring, as it reflected a greater attentiveness: straighter posture, eyes that were alert. The question was whether improved student attitudes could lead to greater academic and, later, professional success.

The good news from the instructor's point of view was that students became less anonymous to her as she began to see "thinking skills" made evident in their journals and buddy exchanges. The experience was much the same as that of Ruth R. Voigniet (1995) who wrote:

> I learned things from the writing that I had never seen before. It was almost possible to 'get inside of the students' minds.' It was possible to tell when they did not truly understand what they were being asked to describe. We could see problems in critical thinking where a student made a judgment based on insufficient or incomplete information. (Proceedings #10)

The students themselves had a different perspective. At the end of the semester they declared they had found micro-themes, listing, brainstorming, free writing, and comparisons to be particularly effective in enhancing thinking and learning. They also indicated in personal interviews with a disinterested (non-faculty) interviewer that they felt more inclined to participate in class than they had at the outset, more intellectually involved, more positive about their learning than they had been in the beginning. They were less anxious about writing and more confident of their ability to succeed. Their positive attitudes were confirmed by their grades: the attrition rate of those enrolled in the writing section of Nursing 114 was only 13%, as opposed to the usual 50%.

After three years of refining the writing-to-learn assignments and three individual course evaluations, it was time to make a general assessment of the impact of the new approach. In addition to the anecdotal information provided by students and instructors, perhaps quantifiable data could provide an additional means of understanding its effectiveness. Finding the right method posed problems, however. As Sarah Freedman (1991) points out in "Evaluating Writing," an entirely satisfactory method of determining the effectiveness of instruction either by large-scale testing or classroom assessment is yet to be found (p. 3). Identifying, isolating, and defining the reasons for attitudinal improvement is problematic, and the degree to which they impact student work is even more resistant to measurement. In short, drawing valid conclusions from a situation filled with variables, that is, classrooms, proved to be exceedingly difficult.

In the end, the general evaluation was carried out using three key instruments: a Writing-to-Learn Attitudinal Survey (WTLAS) administered in a pretest-posttest design, scheduled interviews, and final course grades (see Table 8.1). They provided evidence of several significant effects of using writing-to-learn techniques in the nursing classroom. Specifically, they confirmed that such strategies (1) improved student attitudes toward writing and learning, (2) strengthened student-teacher communication, and (3) increased student retention (Dobie & Poirrier, 1996).

On the first day of a new semester the WTLAS, based on other similar surveys, classroom writing histories, and Daly and Miller's (1975) writing apprehension test, was administered to the 131 students enrolled in Nursing 114. At the end of the term, following administration of a wide variety of writing-to-learn activities dealing with nursing theories and trends, as well as ethical, stressful, and legal issues, the same Writing-to-Learn Attitudinal Survey was administered as a posttest. Composed of nine negative and twenty-one positive statements about writing, it was designed to cover basic psychosocial apprehensions and positive and negative perceptions about writing. It provided a means for categorizing data in terms of positive and negative differences in attitudes and perceptions about writing.

To analyze the data provided by the WTLAS, the paired t-test (alpha = .05) was used to determine the significance of differences between pretest and posttest scores. It revealed that students

Table 8.1
Writing-to-Learn Attitudinal Survey
Pretest/Posttest

The College of Nursing is trying to determine the effectiveness of using writing to improve student learning and success. Would you please complete the following survey to help us gather information that will be important in designing courses for other students?

Name: _____

Student ID Number: _____

Course: _____

Date: _____

Below are a series of statements about writing. There are no right or wrong answers to these statements. Please indicate the degree to which each statement applies to you by marking the appropriate number on the Scantron form with a pencil as follows: (1) strongly agree, (2) agree, (3) uncertain, (4) disagree, or (5) strongly disagree with the statement. While some of these statements may seem repetitious, take your time and try to be as honest as possible.

STRONGLY AGREE	AGREE	UNCERTAIN	DISAGREE	STRONGLY DISAGREE
1	2	3	4	5

1. Expressing ideas through writing seems to be a waste of time.
2. Impromptu focused writing in class helps me to solve problems or clarify concepts.
3. I get nervous when I am asked to write.
4. Handing in written questions about lectures and reading assignments helps me understand course material.
5. I like to write my ideas down.
6. I feel confident in my ability to express my ideas clearly in writing.
7. Informal notes and letters to classmates about course material help me to understand difficult material.
8. I enjoy writing.
9. Brainstorming, freewriting, or listing ideas before writing helps me find out what I know and think about a topic.
10. I have a terrible time organizing my ideas in writing.
11. Admit slips make it easier to begin thinking about what will be covered in a class.
12. I like seeing my thoughts on paper.
13. I avoid writing if possible.
14. I would enjoy submitting my writing to magazines for evaluation and publication.
15. I like to have my friends read what I have written.
16. I never seem to be able to write my ideas down clearly.
17. Writing micro-themes (brief summaries) makes me aware of the most important points in reading assignments.
18. I don't think I write as well as most people.
19. Critiquing a classmate's writing for conceptual clarity results in increased understanding for both of us.
20. Writing personal experience pieces makes me see connections between what I am learning and my own life.
21. I'm no good at writing.
22. Writing to different audiences makes me aware of how much the reader or listener affects the way I state information and concepts.
23. Good writers make better grades in college than poor writers.
24. It's easy for me to express my ideas in writing.
25. The technical aspects of writing (punctuation, spelling, etc.) are more important than other aspects (concept formulation, clarity, etc.).
26. I don't like my writing to be evaluated.
27. Writing skills are necessary for success.
28. Exit slips help me to remember the main points covered in a class.
29. Discussing my writing with others is an enjoyable experience.
30. I use journals to enhance my understanding of course materials.

responded more positively to the statements on the WTLAS as a posttest, that is, after they had experienced the writing activities, than they did as a pretest. The scores on the pretest and posttest were significantly different ($t = 9.17$, $p = .0001$). For example, 45% of the students stated on the pretest that they were nervous when asked to write, but only 35% confessed to such feelings on the posttest.

The second phase of evaluation took place two weeks before the end of the semester when a graduate student (not previously involved in the study) conducted twenty-minute interviews with twenty students who volunteered to act as representatives of the class. The conversations were carried out for two purposes: to confirm or dispute the findings of the WTLAS and to discover information not revealed by it. The interviewer queried the students about their responses to the in-class writings: Were they helpful in learning course material? In understanding it and using it? Did the students use the writing techniques in other course work? Did they become more personally involved with their profession through writing about it? Which activities were the most helpful? Which were least helpful?

The answers (taped and later transcribed) were generally positive, indicating that the students had found their writing experiences to have assisted their learning. They recognized the importance of writing both in their academic work and in their future careers. Typical of their comments were: "In the process of writing, you find out what you know." "I like to be able to give the accurate answer—if you say what you know, it's more beneficial than A,B,C." "[I] preferred essay and writing exams because I got to write down everything I know, everything I learned."

The third evaluation was carried out at the end of the term when final course grades were compared with those of students in another class taught without the writing interventions. The comparison, confirming a similar one carried out the first year of the pilot program, provided dramatic evidence of differences between the two. The attrition rate for the writing intensive classes ran at 27% as compared to 49% in a section of the same course taught in the traditional manner. Although proving a direct relationship between the writing activities and a higher retention rate may not be possible, it seems likely that the improved student attitudes reflected in the WTLAS and the active involvement called for were strong influences in student commitment and success.

The effects of the new "cognitive approach" were also felt in some surprising areas—not the least of which was the faculty. As the director of writing worked with teachers in nursing, a new cross-disciplinary collegiality developed. They began to recognize common goals and the adaptability of teaching techniques. They realized that despite the dissimilarity of their disciplines, they had much to teach each other about students and learning. The nursing faculty, aware that it had a rich body of information for examining not only teaching strategies, but course content and curriculum as well, began to reassess its offerings. Later they would share their conclusions and applications with faculty in history, English, art, and business, that is, with colleagues across the curriculum.

Teacher-student relationships in nursing were also affected by the inquiry stance of the new approach. As students confronted hard questions that led to other, harder questions, the faculty became more inquiry oriented as well. Urged to write when their students wrote, they found themselves keeping longer and more reflective notes about students, classes, and the profession. To capitalize on this development, and nourish the developing intellectual community, student and faculty volunteers were asked to participate in a mentoring program in which representatives from each group would be paired to research and write articles to be submitted for publication. Twelve students and eight faculty mentors produced seven submitted articles for publication. Five (71%) were accepted for publication in professional nursing journals. Publication had its own unexpected result. Formal participation in professional dialogue through written articles read by practitioners in one's discipline confers power. The ability to put ideas into writing can shape the opinions of others, raise public awareness of issues, and provide information needed to make sound choices. In short, it gives the writer the means to make things happen, or not happen. That skill may be more important now than ever before in the field of nursing.

The instructor's use of writing to facilitate learning and thinking has made its way into other classes, and has even spawned activities (like the Mentoring Project) that do not take place in a class at all. The College of Nursing has made new ties with other departments and faculty in a wide variety of disciplines. Instructors in many universities are discovering the power of making their classrooms places of active learning through student involvement and collaboration, both anchored in the act of writing. They are proving the assertion made by I. A. Richards (1936) over fifty years ago: "Writing defective in logic or grammar or rhetoric short-circuits ideas and prevents their successful functioning. Thus bad writing short-circuits the potentialities of departments, instructors, readers, and students who believe that good writing is a function of good thinking and a continuing force in the process of learning" (p. 12).

We are all learning, whether we teach nursing or art or sociology, that a commitment to writing is a commitment to producing lifelong learners who can think.

REFERENCES

Daly, K. A., & Miller, M. D. (1975). The empirical development of an instrument to measure writing apprehension. *Research in the Teaching of English, 9,* 242–249.

Dobie, A., & Poirrier, G. P. (1996). When nursing students write. *Language and Learning Across the Disciplines, 1*(3), 23–33.

Freedman, S. W. (1991). Evaluating writing: Linking large-scale testing and classroom assessment (Occasional Paper #27). Berkeley, CA: Center for the Study of Writing.

Gere, A. R. (Ed.). (1985). *Roots in the sawdust.* Urbana, IL: National Council of Teachers of English.

McLeod, S. (1987). Defining writing across the curriculum. *WPA: Writing Program Administration, 11*(1–2), 19–24.

Richards, I. A. (1936). *The philosophy of rhetoric.* New York: Oxford University Press.

Voigniet, R. R. (1995). Reflections on the writing of student nurses: Understanding our program and curriculum. In S. Gamboa, C. Lovitt, & A. Williams (Eds.), *Proceedings of the second national conference on writing across the curriculum* (p. 10). Charleston, SC: College of Charleston.

Chapter Nine

WRITING EXPERIENCES IN THE DEVELOPMENT OF PROFESSIONAL NURSING ETHICS

Teresa Mumme Margaglio, MS, RN, CS-FNP, IBCLC

*J*unior level nursing students in the baccalaureate program of the university consider legal, ethical, and political issues involved in nursing during a two-credit hour course. Because the students are beginning their clinical rotations, the course offers them an opportunity to begin developing their professional nursing ethics which will guide them in their practice of nursing. The course is designed to encourage the students to consider their personal values as a basis for professional decision making and to progress to the recognition of their role in healthcare for the community through political responsibility. Specific writing-to-learn activities are incorporated throughout the course to assist nursing students with ethical, legal, and political role development.

Upon completion of this course, the student should be able to demonstrate an understanding of the concept of caring as a basis for their nursing activities and to consider ethical decisions from a caring perspective. The students are afforded opportunities to review and analyze ethical thinking processes and to evaluate methods of formulating defensible resolutions to dilemmas encountered in nursing practice. They should be able to discuss resolutions to ethical dilemmas and evaluate resolutions to ethical decisions encountered in nursing practice from legal, moral, ethical, and political perspectives.

The students are requested to consider their personal and professional philosophy as their first writing experience for the course. They consider their personal beliefs through the process of introspection and are asked to articulate these beliefs as a basis for their living will declaration. The living will should reflect the wishes of the individual and provide a person with the right to self-determination. To assure that personal wishes are followed, a durable power of attorney should be made to insure that someone who knows the individual's wishes will see that they are followed if the person is unable to make decisions for themselves. Sharing these wishes through clearly articulated personal and philosophical ideas with family and friends will protect the right of self-determination.

Students are asked to include the following areas in their personal philosophies: their health, the importance of relationships, their attitudes toward life: (hobbies, recreation, fears, joys, dreams, etc.), their attitudes toward personal illness and dying, the illness or dying of their significant others, and death in general. They are asked to write a brief statement of their professional philosophy including five of their professional values and their significance to them. Writing and articulating personal beliefs help to raise the consciousness of the individual right of self-determination. Acting to protect this right for others is the basis for nursing ethics.

Students move from personal issues to current ethical issues that are found in daily newspapers. The students are asked to select an issue, take an ethical position, and formulate their arguments. The students are asked to select at least two solutions and predict the consequences of each solution. These positions are presented in small groups and the process used is evaluated by their peers. Considering current issues increases individual awareness of ethical dilemmas in daily living.

The students submit a formal library research paper that is expected to succinctly and clearly present an ethical, legal, or political issue that includes applications to nursing practice. Students grade their own papers before submitting them, utilizing guidelines that help the students to focus on scholarly presentation and correct usage of the APA format. Faculty members grade and comment on the quality and clarity of the research presentation. Correct grammar, punctuation, and spelling and accurate documentation of references are expected throughout the paper. Students also give formal verbal presentations to the class. These presentations are graded on the student's organization and familiarity with material, and clarity in presentation without reading notes. Presentations allow the students to share their research and findings with their peers. Clarity and organization of presentations are influenced by the level of research and construction of the written paper.

The final writing experience for the students is sending correspondence to their congressman. Political activity begins with the recognition that the individual has a responsibility for and a voice in the legislation that is enacted. Legislation affects the individual, the profession of nursing, the community, the environment, and the world. Voting is the first level of political responsibility and activity that requires individuals to take a stand on the election of politicians and legislative issues. After affecting the political milieu through exercising the right to vote, individuals need to express their beliefs and wishes, instruct politicians on issues and health needs of the community, and express support for the position taken by the politician on issues of interest to the individual. Students recognize the need for writing legislators when they receive personal responses to their own comments and positions.

A variety of writing experiences are utilized in the course to help students clarify their thought processes regarding a new experience in learning. The processes of ethical decision making can be taught in class. The actual understanding of ethics needs to be a process of introspection and clarification through the articulation of personal values. Utilization of ethical theories in the decision-making process helps students to recognize the resolution of issues and to distinguish between knowledge, fact, and values. Participation in the process of corresponding with legislators may open avenues of political activity that remain active during professional careers.

Chapter Ten

Computer Writing in Nursing

Carolyn Delahoussaye, DNS, RN
Gail P. Poirrier, DNS, RN

*C*omputer technology has far reaching implications for nursing practice and professional nursing education. Nurses are required to use computer technology to develop and implement the nursing process, to engage in clinical research activities, to advance their own accountability and nursing knowledge, and to provide educational information to consumers of healthcare. Utilization of computer technology provides nursing practice with new methods for data collection, comprehensive documentation, interactive networking, communication, accessing national and international information about current healthcare practice, storage of health information, reception and dissemination of information, and internal and cost effective management.

The challenge to incorporate computer technology within professional nursing programs has been mandated. The Healthy People 2000 (Mason, 1990) initiative has set as a priority the systematic collection, analysis, interpretation, dissemination, and use of health data in planning preventive programs to protect the health status of the population of the United States. Education for healthcare professionals calls for increased attention to computer technology which increases access to information. The National League for Nursing (1992a) supports change in educational methods to a community-centered technology-based teaching format and views use of computer technology as critical to this change.

Utilization of computer technology assists students with critical thinking and communication skills. Computer technology is simply a tool rather than the focus. An individual's intellect, thinking, and communication skills are the basis for utilization of computer technology. ". . . technology assists people and supplements their basic capabilities. The individual remains accountable and responsible" (Simpson, 1994, p. 271).

The use of computer technology in nursing includes one's ability to write and communicate in a manner that is supported by critical thinking skills. Computerized writing skills are necessary in practice. Nurses utilize computer systems for communication purposes such as: writing nursing care plans, expanding one's nursing knowledge base, networking with professional and accrediting nursing organizations, dissemination of research findings, and critiquing computer software for continuing education and clinical use. Writing via computer technology gives the opportunity to healthcare workers to communicate information to other healthcare professionals at various work sites such as rural and specialty clinics, home health agencies, home health client environments, schools, hospitals, professional education institutions, etc. By incorporating computer technology within professional nursing education curricula, graduates will be better prepared to communicate as a team member with other healthcare workers to enhance integration of health services, manage and use patient information data, and disseminate client-focused healthcare information within the context of community needs.

The following is an example of how computer technology can be incorporated into a professional nursing curriculum across levels. The project, a computer portfolio, was developed as a response to the National League for Nursing (1992b) Required Outcome Criterion 2: Communication which reflects student abilities in the areas of communication and information technology. The purpose of the computer portfolio was to enhance written communication and critical thinking skills through a variety of computer technology applications relevant to curriculum level content. Student learning outcomes related to computer technology were developed for each baccalaureate clinical nursing course, a senior nursing computer course, and a bridge course in the BSN degree completion program for licensed nurses. The computer technology objectives are the same across the curriculum for all clinical nursing courses. These are:

1. Use information resources and information-handling tools to support person, scholarly, and practice activities.
2. Use a variety of computer hardware and software for instructional, research, and practice purposes.
3. Maintain integrity and security of data files.

Computer assignments were developed to meet the above objectives and vary within courses and levels according to the clinical focus.

The first clinical course in nursing is offered at the sophomore level. Students enrolled in this course are oriented to the computer portfolio at the beginning of the semester. The portfolio is actually begun at this level, added to at each subsequent level, and must be completed prior to admission into the senior level computer nursing course, Computer Applications in Nursing. Each student develops their own portfolio which provides documentation of computer writings that meet various communication and critical thinking objectives within each clinical nursing course. All student portfolios are housed in one central location under the direction of the faculty of record for the Computer Applications in Nursing course. Each semester, students within all courses must complete and turn in the appropriate computer assignment documentation for that semester. There are no letter grades attached to this specific course requirement, however, the portfolios are assessed for satisfactory completion of the computer objectives. This requirement must be achieved before students can receive their awarded course grade.

At the sophomore level, students are oriented to the College of Nursing computer lab during a one-hour orientation period. Students must sign up for these orientation periods outside of actual class time. The computer lab staff orient the students to the computer as well as to word processing and are available throughout the semester for assistance to students for computer related needs. The sophomore nursing course syllabus contains a short tutorial in using word processing and students are encouraged to purchase other word processing guides. This early orientation to computers assists students to begin using computer technology at the start of their clinical nursing education.

Although the University provides students with an orientation to the university library, students forget. They still need to be oriented to specific areas related to nursing. Initially it was left to students to get oriented by themselves. Negotiations with library support personnel brought about a shared work. The library provides a packet of printed information for each student explaining all available resources. At the beginning of the semester, the librarian attends the students' class and hands out the packets as well as provides an in-depth orientation to library services that particularly meet the needs of nursing students throughout their professional education.

The assignments for the computer portfolio at the sophomore level involve using a word processing program for each assignment. Students may use the computers in the College of Nursing computer lab or any computer software which they have access to. All assignments must include student name, course number, and date. Each assignment is limited to one printed page.

1. Search LIBIS (library computerized catalog system)
    a. Use the university library computerized catalogue system (LIBIS) to access two nursing related books.
    b. Report all bibliographical information as well as the call numbers and the number of copies available in the university library.
2. Literature Database Search
    a. Use the library CDRom electronic database to do a nursing research literature database search.
    b. Write a brief description of your selections including all bibliographical information and a synopsis of the abstract.
3. Computer-Assisted Instruction (CAI) Critique
    a. Select two CAI programs required by your nursing course.
    b. Provide a written critique of each program including the following: name and type (problem solving, drill and practice, tutorials, simulation) of CAI, completion time, completeness of directions, comments regarding screen design.

The library computer assignments assist beginning clinical nursing students to focus on such course content as relating research findings to specific nursing actions for individual clients, applying concepts and theories from the sciences and humanities, and relating nursing roles to the health needs of individual patients. If students are to be successful in a fast paced, heavy content based curriculum, a working understanding of library computer technology is a must for knowledge comprehension, expansion and application. The written CAI critique enhances critical thinking and communication skills. Examples of CAI programs that relate specifically to critical thinking and communication skills and designed for basic or fundamental nursing content include Using the Nursing Process, Nursing Decision Making, and Nurse Patient Interaction.

Students enrolled in first semester junior, second semester junior and first semester senior clinical nursing courses have the following assignments:

1. Computer-Assisted Instruction (CAI) Critique
   a. Select two CAI programs required by your nursing course.
   b. Provide a written critique of each program including the following: name and type (problem solving, drill and practice, tutorials, simulation) of CAI, completion time, completeness of directions, comments regarding screen design.
2. Nursing Care Plan
   a. Create a nursing care plan for a client you have cared for during this semester. Include: Data Cues, Nursing Diagnosis, Expected Outcomes/Client Goals, Nursing Actions and Evaluation headings.
   b. Use a word processing columns/table format.

Examples of CAI programs that enhance critical thinking and communication skills are listed for each of the upper level clinical courses:

1. First Semester Junior Course
   a. Eliminating Pediatric Medication Errors
   b. Nursing Pediatric Nursing Series

    c. Pharmacologic Interventions in Obstetrical Care

    d. The Wills: A Neonate and His Young Adult Mother

    e. 12-Point Postpartal Check

2. Second Semester Junior Course

    a. Mr. Carl, A Young Adult Undergoing an Ileostomy

    b. Nursing Decisions: A Postoperative Patient

    c. Mr. Kane, an Adult Experiencing Respiratory Syndrome

3. First Semester Senior Course

    a. A Patient in Cardiogenic Shock

    b. Two Patients with MI

    c. A Patient with CHF and Pulmonary Edema

Computer care-plan writing helps students to focus on the critical care components for given patients as assigned in each clinical nursing course. This assignment assists the students to demonstrate through computer writing their roles as caregiver, advocate, health teacher, leader, researcher, collaborator, and change agent as they apply the nursing process to care of patients with obstetrical, pediatric, and medical-surgical health needs. This assignment also mandates that students learn a computer skill, such as creating tables, and writing and editing within tables. This form of computer writing gives the students an opportunity to engage in a type of writing that is required for documentation in nursing practice.

Satisfactory completion of all computer portfolio documents is the prerequisite for enrollment in Computer Applications in Nursing that is offered during the final semester of the senior year. During this course, students continue to add to the portfolio. All university students have access to the Internet via the university mainframe computer. Students enrolled in nursing are required to activate their mainframe account at the beginning of the course. This is a free service. Once all accounts have been activated, students are oriented to various aspects of the Internet including E-mail, gopher, Archie, Veronica, and web browsing.

The first assignment requires each student to send an E-mail message to the instructor providing the instructor with the student's

E-mail address. This E-mail message is placed in the student's computer portfolio. The instructor then sends an acknowledgment to each student. Students must save the message to a file and print the file. This printed sheet is placed in the student's computer portfolio. Thereafter, all assignments are sent to students via E-mail. Requiring students to utilize E-mail in this manner enhances the students' communication skills. The assignment focuses on clarity of communication. In addition, it gives the students an opportunity to experience current state-of-the-art computer communication systems.

The class is divided into small groups of 3 to 4 students per group. Each group is assigned a topic related to computer use in nursing. Topics include: History of Healthcare Computing, Hospital and Nursing Information Systems, Clinical Practice Applications: Institution and Community-Based, Research and Education Applications, Confidentiality, Ergonomics, and Nursing Informatics Education. Each group must use some type of electronic search to find at least two research articles on their topic. Groups then do a class presentation and provide their classmates with complete bibliographic references and content outlines of the research. This assignment builds on computer writing skills learned at the sophomore level. At this advanced level, students are now using computer writing to share information with classmates. This enhances critical thinking and clarity of course content. In addition, this assignment mandates that the graduating senior focus on the importance of research in education and practice.

Another assignment is to develop a professional vita for use in obtaining employment. This must be done on a computer and students are encouraged to be as creative as they wish. This assignment enhances professional growth and development.

The final assignment is designed to assist students in gaining knowledge about nurse practice acts across the United States. This enhances professional growth and development, increases their nursing knowledge related to legalities and public policies that impact nursing practice, and allows them to access information pertinent to nursing practice via the computer. Each student is assigned a specific state and must use the Internet to search for the nurse practice act of their assigned state. The report that is handed in provides a detailed roadmap of where they traveled on the Internet to find the information as well as a copy of the act downloaded from the Internet site. If the information is not available on the Internet, then the student is responsible for submitting a roadmap as well as contacting the state board of nursing for verification that the practice act is not available on the Internet.

Upon graduation, each student's completed computer portfolio contains evidence of the following computer writings: library searches, computer assisted instruction critiques, nursing care plans, E-mail communications, research information files, professional vitae, and documents via the Internet. Graduates express gratitude for the computer experience while a student. Graduate exit surveys reflect that students feel prepared to utilize computers in clinical practice as well as in future personal and professional growth experiences. Future plans include updated additions to computer assignments and follow up of students' continued or expanded computer use after graduation.

REFERENCES

Mason, J. O. (1990). *Healthy people 2000: National health promotion and disease prevention objectives* (DHHS Publication No. PHS91-50213). Washington, DC: U.S. Government Printing Office.

National League for Nursing. (1992a). *An agenda for nursing education reform—In support of nursing's agenda for health care reform.* New York: NLN Press.

National League for Nursing. (1992b). *Criteria and guidelines for the evaluation of baccalaureate and higher degree programs in nursing.* New York: NLN Press.

Simpson, R. L. (1994). The computer-based patient record and how it will affect the nurse's practice. In J. McCloskey, & H. Grace (Eds.), *Current issues in nursing* (4th ed., pp. 270–275). St. Louis: Mosby.

Chapter Eleven

TECHNICAL WRITING—
NURSING DOCUMENTATION

Peggy A. McCabe, RN, MSN
Susan M. Randol, RN, MSN

Nursing students must learn a discipline-specific form of communication—nursing documentation. This form of writing provides the documentation of care provided to their clients. Nursing documentation supplies the validation that standards of care are accomplished and allows for the billing of services provided to the client. This documentation is a communication skill that requires a significant amount of practice. Nursing documentation is taught in the beginning nursing courses and learning and practice continues throughout the remainder of the nursing curriculum. Students have been introduced to documentation through the use of textbooks, class lectures, and actual practice in the past. Interaction with a clinical information system is another method for learning documentation which has become available.

The JRS Clinical Information System (JRS-CIS) is a computer system that includes a documentation system for nurses. It offers an effective, efficient way to communicate a nurse's findings and actions. Computers, a frightening concept for many nurses and student nurses, are not what they traditionally think of in conjunction with nursing, at least, not when it comes to the all important documentation. From the beginning, the JRS-CIS was expected to serve a number of purposes when used with nursing students. Four of the purposes are as follows: (1) introduce computers to beginning level nursing students, (2) facilitate accurate and thorough nursing communication, (3) emphasize the need for nurses to communicate with other nurses and members of other disciplines, and (4) to assist student nurses with real-world strategies for the provision and documentation of care they provide.

Set Up Clinical Information System

A grant from the FULD foundation provided funds for the purchase of computer hardware and the JRS-CIS (developed by JRS Clinical

Technologies) that is used within the College of Nursing at the University of Southwestern Louisiana. The JRS-CIS is being used by numerous hospitals across the United States. The version of the JRS-CIS purchased uses a UNIX operating system therefore a standalone server was purchased for storage and use of the system. (This is the only UNIX-based software the College of Nursing has purchased for use on its system.) The system is set up to use the cable put in for the College of Nursing Local Area Network (LAN) and the University's network. There are approximately 40 to 50 (20 student, 20 to 30 faculty) personal computers (PCs) that are able to operate using PC-based software or the JRS-CIS.

The JRS-CIS is being customized for each clinical course to use with students. A unit, with the same number of patients as students in the course, is established for the use of students in a particular clinical course. Then a menu with specific activities is prepared based on consultation and decisions made with the master teacher for the clinical course. The unit and menu are accessible only to the students in the course for which they are developed. Nursing faculty have access to all of the units and menus on the system. Sophomore students learn and are tested on basic nursing skills in the clinical course at their level. When the students are tested on the skills such as vital signs, intake and output measures, mobility, positioning, wound care, and other skills, they go from the testing to a computer terminal and document their findings and/or care on the clinical information system. Each of the skill areas is available on the menu accessible for those sophomore nursing students. The nursing students save their documentation on the particular simulated client assigned and nursing faculty are able to review the work when convenient. Junior nursing students in the Pediatric and Obstetric course document assessment information, obtained on a patient they care for in the hospital, on the clinical information system. The junior students document the information obtained using a simulated client on the unit established for their course in the clinical information system. The documentation of information on a simulated client allows for maintenance of client confidentiality for the client actually provided care in the hospital. Documentation put into the system by the students is saved for faculty review when it is convenient. After the faculty review the documentation, they provide feedback to the students about the documentation. Similar activities are provided for senior students. Progression in the nursing student's computer documentation skill is provided as they progress through the nursing curriculum.

The clinical information system is set up for users to select their documentation from a list of common terms or conditions for each area or system for documentation. When there is no selection that works for the client situation or condition there is an ability to create and save narrative notes which describe the situation or condition. This allows the students to be accurate with their communication of information. Menu selections related to documentation of the client's general condition and safety were left on for sophomore nursing students to view though they are not specifically tested on those areas in the skills lab. This provides an example for the sophomore nursing students to learn about the types of information that would be included in the communication about the client's general condition and safety.

IMPLEMENTATION

The JRS-CIS is being introduced at the sophomore level with the first clinical course. This is the basic fundamentals course that is taught in conjunction with a physical assessment course. There are usually 80 to 90 students in the courses who come with varied backgrounds and experiences in nursing and computers use. The first semester the JRS-CIS was introduced an informal show of hands on the first day of class indicated that over half of the students did not have computer experience and/or did not have access to computers.

The many possibilities for computer access were explained to the students including the College of Nursing student computer lab. There are two full-time computer support staff in the lab for help at any time. Times were set up at the beginning of the semester for a short course on how to use the computers and available software. The JRS-CIS system was not explained at that time due to time constraints. This was strictly to familiarize the students with computers and how to operate them and was essential for further use of the system.

The first six weeks of the basic fundamentals course is used to introduce, learn, and test important basic nursing skills, such as vital signs, bed baths/linen change, range of motion, transfers from beds to wheelchairs, and sterile dressing changes, to name a few. These tasks and the assessment findings that go along with any patient contact must be documented. The problem was how to teach and test 80+ students on nursing basics and also have them document their findings on the computer with no additional time available.

Each semester the students are divided into three groups, each coming on a different day for demonstrations, practice, and skills testing. All of the 3 to 4 faculty would participate in these activities. It was decided to use one of the faculty in the computer lab exclusively. The two computer support staff, who are not nurses, were unable to block the time needed each week just for this exercise. Five computers were used simultaneously by the students. An initial orientation was given on getting into the system from the main menu. The students finished testing in the skills lab and went directly to the computer lab where they were given their account identifier, password, and patient assignment. They must remember these numbers and these numbers stay with the nursing students until they graduate. They will be required to document certain data and information on that same patient throughout subsequent clinical nursing courses. The account ID and passwords were created so that the students could easily remember them. If the student forgot the information, it is available from one of the system administrators.

The first nursing skills the students learned pertained to mobility needs. Each student was individually walked through each menu and screen pertaining to mobility. These screens listed possible items for documentation, such as turning every hour or 2 hours, what position, assistance required, the condition of the skin, and so on. Students usually do not know the language at this level and had to be instructed on what was important and what should be included. This was the amazing thing about this computer system and what contributed to its success in our program. The terminology was there in front of the student. Each category gave a variety of appropriate choices which would lead to other options for the students. These choices were used as cues by the students. Findings that they had assessed but never realized were important would come up on the screen. At first, the students would question whether the statement was really an important item to record or would express amazement that they had not thought of it themselves. As the physical assessment course which runs in conjunction with the basic fundamentals course proceeded, the students were able to see the connections between some of the statements on the computer system and what findings and aspects of patient care were important. As they progressed through the semester, these cues encouraged them to critically think beyond the level expected by sophomore nursing students.

After two sessions on the computer the students made excellent progress using the JRS-CIS for communication of information. Because the skills and the language were still new to them the instructor remained close to answer questions pertaining to nursing. Use of the system techniques for documentation were mastered by this time. The students had only one computer use problem which was when the JRS-CIS system was not on screen. They had to go through several menus to get to the JRS-CIS which allowed the inexperienced computer users to get lost. The computer staff solved this by composing simple instructions and posting them on each computer used for documentation on the JRS-CIS. The students with little computer experience then mastered the system quickly.

The large numbers of students seen in the computer lab seemed daunting at first. At least 30 were seen each day, but there were only five students (a manageable number) working on the documentation system at a time. Students could be counseled individually as they progressed at their own speed through the menus and screens. They could also easily be addressed as a small group. The computer support staff was always on hand for computer questions and difficulties.

OUTCOMES

The positive outcomes from using this computer system and starting at this level were apparent both to the nursing faculty and to the students. Since the students learned the terminology early in the course they were familiar with it by the time they went into the clinical setting. The faculty immediately noticed a difference between these students knowledge and abilities in assessments and charting and those of students from previous semesters. These students were more organized in their thought processes, they assessed the whole patient and looked at possibilities for assessment or comfort measures beyond the scope of a student at this level. Also, the students had very positive comments about their experience with documentation using JRS-CIS. They continually expressed amazement while using the system about the scope of nursing and areas important for documentation. They said they never realized nurses looked at the comfort measures, the psychological aspects, and the indepth assessment parameters. Many were under the impression that nurses only perform tasks and follow orders and did not realize that nurses look at the whole person and think for themselves. The students also stated that they felt more comfortable in the clinical setting and felt more secure in what they were able to offer their patients. Several stated that they really thought about patient comfort overall instead of just in relation to the task performed.

Use of this computer system enhanced the learning capabilities of these beginning level nursing students. They learned the importance of accurate and thorough communication. The system also prepared them for real world situations in computer use and it expanded their abilities to critically think. Becoming familiar with the terminology and language of nursing made them more confident and better able to care for their patients, especially at the beginning level.

Chapter Twelve

WRITING TO ENHANCE RESEARCH

A COLLABORATIVE PROJECT WITH PRACTICING NURSES

Evelyn M. Wills, PhD, RN

Writing-to-learn strategies are adaptable to the process of learning to critique research. Graduates of baccalaureate nursing programs are expected to be informed consumers of nursing research and to be able to critique research reports for use in clinical practice (Burns & Grove, 1995). The writing-intensive method of instruction in critical thinking is an excellent vehicle for guiding students in learning to critique research. Strategies of critical thinking include comparing research findings to a set of external criteria that are accepted throughout the scientific community. Baccalaureate prepared nurses appraise research based on evaluation criteria that may have been internalized in an undergraduate research course. Nurses in clinical practice must evaluate research for clinical use with the needs of the institution, its nursing staff, and the patient-consumers in mind (Horne Video Productions, 1991).

Utilization of research in nursing practice is increasingly necessary as funding agencies review the efficacy of nursing interventions and accrediting agencies demand research validation (Joint Commission on Accreditation of Healthcare Organizations [JCAHO], 1995). Students of baccalaureate programs commonly learn the rudiments of the research process in a variety of ways. Traditionally, nursing students were tasked with writing a research proposal. In some curricula, they assist a seasoned researcher in data collection, some curricula have students read research articles in preparing for a clinical practicum, or students are required to critique research articles for clinical utilization (Beyea, Farley, & Williams-Burgess, 1996; Halloran, 1996; Overfield & Duffy, 1984). The current role of the baccalaureate nursing student in research has been redefined as that of informed consumer of research (Burns & Grove, 1995; National League for Nursing [NLN], 1992).

Evaluation is an abstract process based on a high-level educational objective (Bloom, 1956). Students are frequently confused as to how to fulfill the objectives of the course. Faculty find themselves teaching research to students who believe research is abstract, mystifying or dry, uninteresting, and of limited use in practice (Halloran, 1996; Kee & Rice, 1995). Bringing the research process to students in interesting ways and presenting them with a positive picture of the research process is a challenge. Recently, nursing educators have developed new, student-learning-centered, rather than research-process-centered ways of teaching research (Beyea, Farley, & Williams-Burgess, 1996; Floyd, 1996; Halloran, 1996; Kee & Rice, 1995; Kessenich, 1996; Pond & Bradshaw, 1996).

An effective nursing research course focuses on coaching students to critique research reports using accepted criteria, to focus on research that is usable within a chosen clinical practice area, to critique the research based on the needs of the nurses and patients in the clinical unit, and to predict the usefulness of the research to patient care in the setting in which the student is currently practicing.

Pond and Bradshaw (1996) and Miller (1996), working independently, studied the attitudes of baccalaureate nursing students using teaching strategies in which students participated in critiquing and disseminating research with practicing nurses. Both found that participation by students in the research endeavor, whether from the standpoint of assisting with data collection (Pond & Bradshaw, 1996) or by presenting a critical appraisal of a research article to practicing nurses (Miller, 1996) improved students' attitudes toward research and contributed to their ultimate ability to use the research process.

Payne and McCabe (personal communication, March 20, 1993) compared teaching research critique using computer-assisted instruction with the didactic (lecture-discussion) method to a group of students composed of generic baccalaureate nursing students, second-degree seeking nursing students, and baccalaureate-completion registered and licensed practical nursing students. Students selected which method—computer-assisted instruction or lecture/discussion—they would use for learning research. The two groups using different methods experienced no significant differences in the final class average for either segment of the research classes over a period of three years (Payne &

McCabe, 1993, unpublished report of internally funded Educational Improvement Mini Grant).

Based on the experiences of several authors and Payne and McCabe, the research course was redesigned to focus on critique of research using videos (Horn Video Productions, 1991) and computer-assisted instruction (CAI) (Castles, 1989) as the instructional method for the basic information and research process. Seminars in critique of research were held at regular intervals throughout the semester to demonstrate the critiquing process and to give students an opportunity to practice the process.

The process of critiquing nursing research is not a single-stage activity, rather, critiquing nursing research is a multistage process that demands that the student learn:

1. The basics of the research process;
2. How to apply the accepted criteria for excellent research to the report at hand;
3. Research must produce outcomes that are acceptable to patients, to the nurses, and to the hierarchy of the institution;
4. How to apply criteria that become evident only from working within an institution.

In the first phase, students learn the criteria for excellence in research by learning the steps of the research process. This is done through computer-assisted instruction (CAI). The second phase involves review of the steps of research and initiation into the research utilization process using the Horn (1991) videos and through seminars in which applying the criteria to research at hand is modeled. The third phase, application of outcomes, is woven through the course in seminars and as one of the course activities. The fourth stage, discriminating institutional and practicing nurse criteria is learned much later in the process, although the students begin working with practicing nurses to learn their needs during this course. Students in the fourth phase of critiquing research learn that it is necessary to apply criteria to research that are acceptable to practicing nurses in a given institution. Through discussions in seminar, students come to realize that the needs of nurses and the consumers of healthcare may differ among institutions or practice settings.

Critiquing research articles for their usefulness in practice makes the rather esoteric process of research meaningful to nursing students (Miller, 1996). To build the research critiquing process into a living experience, these senior nursing students were required to meet with practicing nurses in their current clinical rotations. Groups of students conferred with the nurses at the clinical sites to develop an understanding of what research the practicing nurses needed that might be available in their specific field of interest. The students then obtained research articles that addressed the topics of interest of their nurse colleagues.

In several seminars throughout the semester, students in self-chosen groups were assigned to read additional research articles as a class activity. The specific research articles were chosen using the clinical course's class schedule for their relevance to the students' current clinical rotation and the content in the clinical nursing course they were attending. The focus of the research process for the unit was the part of the article being critiqued during the seminar. For instance, if the topic of discussion was critique of the problem statement, question, and hypothesis, student groups would focus on identifying those elements of the research report and applying the critiquing criteria for the element. The study group would choose a speaker to deliver the comments of the group in a scholarly reporting style at the end of each exercise.

Early in the semester, students were encouraged to make contact with practicing nurses in their clinical rotations or with nurses working where they were in practice if they were LPNs or RN to BSN students. Through contact with practicing nurses, the student groups identified an area of research interest and topic for study. The faculty assisted the students in identifying a research article that would be interesting and useful in the practice site they had chosen. Faculty worked with the student groups throughout the semester to coach them in use of criteria in critiquing research reports.

The students' major group project was to write a research critique of no more than ten pages using criteria printed in the syllabus. Students were required to submit a rough draft within two weeks prior to the date of submission of the final critique. A faculty member coached the student groups through written comments on the draft and through personal meetings with the student groups. In most cases, the student's final paper was an example of a research article critiqued in a scholarly manner and giving weaknesses and strengths of the research, recommendations for use clinically, or the need for further testing.

At the end of the semester, the students made a user-friendly handout for their practicing nurse colleagues, developed a presentation of no more than 15 to 20 minutes in length in which they discussed their critique of the research with the nurses, and completed the process with an evaluation of the presentation by the nurses. The user-friendly handout was duplicated and submitted with the final course term paper—the indepth critique. Finally, a presentation was prepared for and given to the class. The members of the class evaluated the presentations of another group by a random drawing process.

Research critique is an excellent medium for students to practice critical thinking and writing. When students are exposed to practicing nurses who require research in their practice arenas and to research that tests and refines clinical nursing interventions, they conclude that research is not only interesting, but also valuable in nursing practice.

The research articles were matched to the students' current topical outline in their clinical course to give them research to read that had relevance for their current clinical practice. This was to develop an appreciation of the relevance of research to their clinical practice. Finally, their interaction with practicing nurses and the acceptance they received for their work was positive in their evaluation of the role research has in clinical nursing.

Course evaluations during the pilot of this new research teaching strategy indicated that students were positive in their appraisal of this strategy. Further, the well-tested CAI approach for learning the basic processes of research were evaluated as effective by the students. Seminars for practicing research critique were interesting affairs and could become forums for discussion of research process, ethics, and other topics the students chose. Writing to enhance research as a teaching strategy for nursing research is an effective method.

References

American Association of Colleges of Nursing. (1987). Essentials of college and university education for professional nursing. *Journal of Professional Nursing, 3*(1), 54–71.

Beyea, S., Farley, J. K., & Williams-Burgess, C. (1996). Teaching baccalaureate nursing students to use research. *Western Journal of Nursing Research, 18,* 213–218.

Bloom, B. S. (Ed.). (1956). *Taxonomy of educational objectives.* New York: David McKay.

Burns, N., & Grove, S. K. (1995). *Understanding nursing research.* Philadelphia, PA: W. B. Saunders.

Castles, M. R. (1989). *Sofprim computer tutor for students, Version II.* St. Louis, MO: A.S.K. Data Systems.

Floyd, J. A. (1996). An undergraduate research course: Emphasis on research utilization. *Journal of Nursing Education, 35*(4), 185–187.

Halloran, L. (1996). Promoting research consumerism in B.S.N. students. *Western Journal of Nursing Research, 18,* 108–110.

Holzemer, W., Slaughter, R., Chambers, D., Dulock, H., & Paul, S. (1990). *Introduction to research: A computer-based tutorial.* San Francisco: University of California.

Horn Video Productions. (1991). *Research utilization: Reading and critiquing a research report* [Videotape]. Ida Grove, IA: Author. (Order No. 391)

Joint Commission on Accreditation of Healthcare Organizations (JCAHO). (1995). *1996 Comprehensive manual for hospitals.* Oak Brook Terrace, IL: Author.

Kee, C. C., & Rice, M. (1995). Nursing research and nursing practice—teaching the inseparable duo. *Western Journal of Nursing Research, 17,* 227–231.

Kessenich, C. R. (1996). Bringing reality to the research classroom. *Journal of Nursing Education, 35,* 187–188.

Miller, P. (1996). Dissemination and utilization of research: Outcome behaviors at the baccalaureate level. *Journal of Nursing Education, 35,* 175–177.

National League of Nursing. (1992). *Criteria and guidelines for the evaluation of baccalaureate and higher degree programs in nursing.* New York: Author. (Publication No. 15-2474)

Overfield, T., & Duffy, M. E. (1984). Research on teaching research in baccalaureate nursing curricula. *Journal of Advanced Nursing, 9,* 180–196.

Pond, E. F., & Bradshaw, M. J. (1996). Attitudes of nursing students toward research: A participatory exercise. *Journal of Nursing Education, 35,* 182–185.

Chapter Thirteen

WRITING FOR HEALTH PROMOTION AMONG THE GENERAL PUBLIC

Anne B. Broussard, RNC, DNS, FACCE

*W*riting-to-learn assignments can be utilized to help nursing students clarify their thoughts and goals, and also to communicate effectively with each other, their instructors, professional nurses, and with the clients to whom they give care. Introduction to client-nurse communication concepts early in the nursing curriculum can assist students in developing the communication skills required for client teaching. This chapter will describe a writing-to-learn assignment designed for a first-semester junior clinical course in which students write newspaper columns for health promotion among the general public.

Writing newspaper columns for the general public requires that students consider areas of interest to the target audience and choose topics narrow enough to be addressed in brief columns. Topics need to be researched in recent publications or with community-based experts to ensure the accuracy and relevancy of the information and advice given. Students can use some of the same client-nurse communication techniques to write columns that they use to communicate verbally with clients. One of the most important skills is to write at the client's level to ensure understanding, while at the same time to "avoid sounding condescending" (Jarvis, 1996, p. 66).

About half of all adults in the United States function either below a fifth grade level or "are only marginally competent readers" (Barnes, 1992a, p. 99). When the target audience is known to have low literacy skills, it is appropriate that materials be written on a fifth- to sixth-grade level (Barnes, 1992b). Newspaper readers, however, are thought to function at an eighth-grade or higher reading level. Students are therefore advised to keep their writing at about an eighth-grade reading level. Students can be given the following guidelines for writing newspaper columns:

- The column should focus on health and health promotion. Specific medical treatments are not to be addressed unless in a general way related to referral to a physician or other primary care professional.

- Write an interesting introduction to catch the reader's attention.
- Keep sentences and paragraphs short.
- Avoid elaborate constructions and phrases.
- Use the active rather than the passive voice.
- Avoid professional jargon unless it is universally recognized (e.g., "prenatal visits" but not "Rh incompatibility").
- Use lists when appropriate with bullets to set off the points and draw the reader's eye to the column.
- Columns are not to exceed more than 2½ to 3½ double-spaced, typed pages.

METHODS

In the first-semester, junior clinical nursing course focusing on nursing care of children and the childbearing family, students are given the option of completing a written assignment for extra credit (two points added to their final course grade average). Each student must have attained passing grades in the maternity and pediatric course components prior to the addition of the two extra points to the final course average.

The goal of this assignment is to help students communicate health information to the lay public while maintaining or honing writing skills. This goal is consistent with two of the course objectives:

1. *Analyzing* the nurse's role of care giver, advocate, and health teacher in the promotion and maintenance of health and the rehabilitation of the childbearing family and the child, and

2. *Appreciating* the role of the nurse as collaborator in health promotion and health maintenance of the childbearing family and the child.

In addition, it is expected that the students who participate will be more likely to participate in optional writing assignments in subsequent courses.

To participate, students write brief newspaper columns on health-related topics of interest to childbearing families. The columns are submitted to the local newspaper for consideration of publication in the College of Nursing's "Nurses' Notes" column. ("Nurses' Notes" is an effort of the college's public relations committee, and contributions on various topics for this column are solicited from faculty members in the College of Nursing.) The students' columns may also be submitted to their hometown newspapers, and the newsletter editor of a local school-based health clinic has recently requested student columns to publish that would be of interest to their readership.

Figure 13.1

Instructions to Students for Optional Written Assignment for Extra Credit

---

OPTIONAL WRITTEN ASSIGNMENT FOR EXTRA CREDIT

Students may complete an optional written assignment for an extra two points added to their final Nursing 301 grade. **ALL** of the following conditions are to be met:

1. Choose to do the assignment alone or in a group of 2-3 students.

2. Make arrangements with a Nursing 301 faculty mentor to guide you. Faculty reserve the right to limit the numbers of students they mentor to manageable numbers.

3. Inform Dr. A. Broussard, within 5 working days after Exam I, of your intention to participate.

4. Write a column for the USL College of Nursing "Nurses' Notes" in the Lafayette Advertiser on a topic of interest to childbearing families. The column should be well-researched for accuracy. Examples of past "Nurses' Notes" are available in Dr. Broussard's office. You may wish to have Wendy Hellinger, our graduate assistant and English major, critique your writing before submitting it to your faculty mentor. Submit the first draft of your column to your faculty mentor, along with your references, before the first clinical day of the second rotation.

5. The faculty mentor either accepts the column as written or returns the column to the student(s) for revision. Subsequent drafts must be completed in sufficient time to allow the faculty mentor time to critique and then to accept the final draft by the midpoint of the second rotation. The mentor will then notify the course coordinator that the student completed the optional written assignment. The finished work will be submitted to the College of Nursing's Public Relations Committee for possible future publication under the student's byline.

6. The student must have attained passing grades (74) in each component of Nursing 301 (Maternity and Pediatric Nursing) prior to the addition of the extra points to the final course average.

(If you want to do this optional assignment, complete #1 on the "Criteria for Acceptance of Assignment" sheet on the next page, have mentor sign on line of #2, and bring to Dr. Broussard within 5 working days after Exam I, but preferably as soon as possible)

Students who are interested are referred to their course syllabus for guidelines on how to proceed and for deadlines and conditions to be met in order for credit to be awarded (Figure 13.1). Students can perform the assignment alone or in groups of two or three, and make arrangements with faculty mentors for guidance. Each student initiates a document from the course syllabus, in order to help the course coordinator track the progress of the par-

Figure 13.2
Documentation of Student Progress in Completing Optional Written Assignment

The University of Southwestern Louisiana
College of Nursing
Department of Baccalaureate Nursing
Nursing 301 - Assignment for Extra Points
Criteria for Acceptance of Assignment

Name of Student:_____

Faculty Signatures (below)	1. Student chose to do assignment: ___ alone ___ with 1-2 other students (names:_____, _____)
	2. Student arranged for faculty mentor. Nursing 301 faculty who agrees to be faculty mentor: _____ (Signature of Nursing 301 faculty member)
(Dr. Broussard) Date:_____	3. Student informed Dr. A. Broussard, within 5 working days after Exam I, of tentative topic: _____, and intention to participate. (Topic)
_____ (Mentor) Date:_____	4. Student submits the first draft, along with references, to mentor before the first clinical day of the second rotation.
_____ (Mentor) Date:_____	5. Final draft, considered by the faculty mentor to be appropriate and well-researched for accuracy, is accepted by the faculty mentor at least by the midpoint of the second rotation.
(Dr. Broussard) Date:_____	The course coordinator is notified of acceptance of student's work -- mentor gives this sheet with column attached to coordinator.
_____ (Dr. Broussard or L. Broussard)	6. The student has attained passing grades (74) in each component of Nursing 301 (Maternity and Pediatric Nursing) prior to the addition of the two extra points to the final course average: Maternity grade_____, Pediatric Nursing grade_____

ticipating students (Figure 13.2). For examples of appropriately written newspaper columns, students have access to past "Nurses' Notes" columns in the course coordinator's office.

Faculty mentors critique the students' writing and work closely with students who need assistance with delineating topics, finding appropriate references, or writing the column. The completed columns are then edited by an in-house graduate assistant in English who has experience writing for newspaper publication. The students receive the edited drafts for further feedback on newspaper-style writing. The finished columns are given to the College of Nursing's Public Relations Committee, which forwards them to the University News Service for submission to the local and/or hometown newspapers for potential future publication under the student's byline.

RESULTS

In the four semesters that this option has been available to students, more than three-fourths of the students finishing the course have completed the assignment, ranging from 57% of the students in the first semester that the option was offered, to 80% to 86% in the last three semesters. The students are encouraged to form groups to write the columns; most of the students work in groups of two or three. Students have little difficulty finding faculty mentors to guide them, since most faculty in the course participate in this activity. Most faculty members who agree to be mentors handle two to three groups a semester; many limit themselves to four groups.

Students have expressed enthusiasm about the assignment and about the opportunity to collaborate with faculty. Faculty mentors have found that a few weeks into the semester, the students are easily able to choose topics and work cooperatively.

Examples of the topics that addressed the needs of the expectant woman or couple and the newborn include:

- Importance of prenatal care.
- Use of different positions for childbirth.
- Paternal-infant bonding.

- Midwifery care as an option for expectant couples.
- Vaginal birth after Caesarean.
- Benefits of breast-feeding.
- Successful breast-feeding techniques.
- Breast-feeding and the working mother.
- Breast-feeding myths.
- Preventing infant deaths due to aspiration.
- Proper sleep positions for the newborn.
- Importance of breast self-exams and mammography.
- Natural childbirth.
- Bottle-mouth syndrome in babies.
- HIV testing in pregnancy.
- Alcohol and pregnancy.
- Physical and psychosocial aspects of adolescent pregnancy.
- Male nurses in the maternity setting.
- Prevention of preterm birth.
- Exercise and pregnancy.
- Smoking and pregnancy.
- Labor and birth in water.
- Postpartal contraception.
- Giving labor support.
- Circumcision.
- Maternal seat belt use.

The needs of parents and children were addressed with topics such as:

- Dealing with the problems of adolescent parenthood.
- Use of hepatitis B virus vaccine.
- Safety seats and seat belts for children.
- Immunizations for children.
- Kidmed services.
- Importance of sex education for children.

- Children at home alone in the summer.
- Munchausen syndrome by proxy.
- Dental health for children.
- Sickle cell disease.
- Childhood allergies.
- Depression in adolescence.
- Protecting toddlers from injuries.
- Pain management in children.
- Play therapy for children.
- Preventing pediatric head injuries.
- Vaccination against chickenpox.
- Swimming lessons and water safety for children.
- Parenting and children's self-esteem.
- Antibiotic therapy for children.
- Ear infections.
- Swimmer's ear.
- Protecting children from sun exposure.

Faculty report that their review of the students' writing and feedback takes a minimal amount of time. Although most students need to revise their first (and sometimes second and third) drafts, students generally have had little difficulty meeting the stated deadlines. Both faculty and students eagerly anticipate the publication of the columns. One example of a published column is illustrated in Figure 13.3 (Dugas, Pons, & Trahan, 1995). It is hoped that the students whose writing is published will feel positive about their efforts and may want to continue their writing and publishing efforts as professional nurses.

Overall, 26.7% of the students completing the optional assignment (20.7% of students completing the course) have received a higher final letter grade in the course as a result (20% to 30% per semester and 16% to 25% per semester, respectively). Students are informed during initial course orientation that completing the assignment has the potential to raise their grade, and many students find this to be a powerful incentive.

Figure 13.3
Example of Published Student News Column

ARE YOUR KIDS HOME ALONE
THIS SUMMER?

by Jamie Dugas, Tracy Pons,
and Hope Trahan
USL Nursing Students

It's summertime, and the kids are out of school. Dad has to work, and Mom does, too. What's a family to do?

Many families this summer will be faced with the problem of child care for the first time. Unfortunately, there are not many affordable summer child care options available for working parents. The only choice some families seem to have is to leave their children at home alone. Such children are commonly known as latchkey children.

Estimates of the number of latchkey children in the United States today range from two to ten million. The greatest risk to such children is their safety. Accidents are the number one cause of death in American children, and latchkey children may be at greater risk for accidents.

While it is not always wise to leave children unattended at home, most experts agree that by age 11, most children are capable of taking care of themselves when they are properly prepared and have demonstrated the ability to follow directions and accept responsibility.

Many latchkey children have not been taught about basic safety or given directions about what to do in an emergency.

Following are some tips to increase a child's safety when he or she must be home alone:
▾ Keep a list of emergency telephone numbers by the telephone. Make certain that your child knows how to report emergencies by dialing 911.

▾ Ask friends or relatives to periodically call and check on your child, if possible.

▾ Give your child a list of telephone numbers of friends or relatives who are likely to be home and available for your child to help with emergencies.

▾ Be certain that your child knows his/her home telephone number, address, and parents' names. Write that information in plain view from the telephone.

▾ Tell your child not to open the door for strangers. Your child may tell callers that his or her parent is taking a bath or shower and cannot come to the door or the telephone.

▾ Teach your child to tell callers that parents are busy. Never tell a caller that parents are not at home. Teach your child to keep doors and windows locked at all times.

▾ Keep a First Aid kit readily available with basic emergency items, and teach your child how to use it.

▾ Instruct your child about proper use of the household appliances that he or she may use while alone.

In addition to ensuring your children's safety, it is also important to provide structured activities for your children. Following are a few ways to keep children well-occupied:

▾ Arrange for specific play times with friends.

▾ Allow times for outside play; make certain rules are understood.

▾ Leave a list of household chores for the child to do.

▾ Rent your child's favorite videos.

▾ Provide a pet as company for your child.

Following these guidelines should help to increase children's safety and decrease parental anxiety about children at home alone.

It has been shown that children can benefit from latchkey experiences by becoming more independent, responsible, and self-reliant. It is the parents' responsibility to prepare and support their children during periods when the children are at home alone.

For more information on child safety, call 232-HELP.

Other incentives include the opportunity to develop collegial relationships with each other and with their faculty mentors, the potential of seeing their writing published, and the opportunity to learn about their role in health promotion as well as to study in depth a chosen content area.

The students' completed columns are arranged each semester into bound booklets in which the students' photographs are included above their respective columns. The booklets are reproduced and distributed to course faculty, the dean and department head, the college student services office, and to all the students in the course. Some of the students have mentioned that they treasure this publication of their work, and are proud to show it to their parents and others.

Nursing care that is directed at health promotion activities will ultimately improve client outcomes and reduce healthcare costs (American Nurses Association, 1991). One way to encourage consumers to be accountable for their own health and to involve themselves in health promotion activities is to reach them through media such as the newspaper. Involvement in writing-to-learn strategies like writing newspaper columns can assist nursing students to assume and develop their roles as health teachers and collaborators in health promotion.

REFERENCES

American Nurses Association. (1991). *Nursing's agenda for health care reform.* Kansas City, MO: Author.

Barnes, L. (1992a). The illiterate client. *MCN, The American Journal of Maternal-Child Nursing, 17*(2), 99.

Barnes, L. (1992b). The illiterate client: Strategies in patient teaching. *MCN, The American Journal of Maternal-Child Nursing, 17*(3), 127.

Dugas, J., Pons, T., & Trahan, H. (1995, June 26). Are your kids home alone this summer? *The Lafayette Advertiser.*

Jarvis, C. (1996). *Physical examination and health assessment* (2nd ed.). Philadelphia, PA: W. B. Saunders.

Chapter Fourteen

VIEWS ABOUT
WRITING-TO-LEARN

Paula C. Broussard, RN, MN

*O*ne of the major complaints about higher education today is class size. Students are requesting smaller classes and more personal learning experiences. Unfortunately, most universities are under mandates to maximize both physical and manpower utilization. The result has been an increased tendency to combine sections into larger classes and even to offer courses via electronic media. Nursing curricula are certainly no exception to these mandates. At the same time nursing programs are attempting to cope with steadily decreasing resources, they are under increasing pressure to provide learning situations that will develop critical thinkers. In its position statement, "Nursing Education's Agenda for the 21st Century," the American Association of Colleges of Nursing identifies processes that are "of critical importance in the student's development of . . . essential cognitive and personal abilities." These processes are critical thinking, information seeking, sorting and selecting, team participation, and critical self-assessment. Nursing faculty are encouraged to establish networks with students that foster role modeling, one-on-one learning strategies, and personal support in the educational process. Further, instructors are directed to carefully monitor and nurture students as they progress through the program (American Association of Colleges of Nursing, 1992). The National League for Nursing's recently revised Criteria for Evaluation of Baccalaureate and Higher Degree Programs explicitly includes critical thinking as a required outcome of nursing education. Specifically, the criterion calls for evidence of "student's skills in reasoning, analysis, research, or decision making relevant to the discipline of nursing" (National League for Nursing, 1992, p. 26).

Upon first consideration, the concepts of financial efficiency with maximum resource utilization and quality instruction that enhances critical thinking appear to be divergent and incongruous ideas. However, creative instructional strategies can help to overcome this apparent incompatibility. Writing-to-learn is certainly one of these creative strategies. One of the most beneficial uses of writing-to-learn concepts is in large classroom situations, when it is all too easy to sacrifice the quality of instruction for the efficiency of enrolling large numbers of students in a single section. Writing offers a way to overcome the impersonal, content-driven situation created by high-enrollment classroom situations. Writing activities get the student more involved in his or her own learning. At the most beneficial level, well-designed writing-to-learn exercises can foster the development of critical thinking by engaging the student in reflection, analytical thinking, and critical analysis.

A cornerstone in the evolution of a critical thinker is the development of reflective thinking. According to Richard Paul (1990), the ability to "think about one's own thinking" is the most essential component of critical thinking. Many writing activities which are perfectly suited to any classroom situation can encourage this kind of thinking.

RELATIONSHIP BETWEEN WRITING AND CRITICAL THINKING

While all thinking is not critical thinking, getting students actively engaged in the learning process and thinking is an important first step. The act of writing necessarily requires thinking on the part of the student. Initially, writing exercises can simply prompt the student to create and organize thoughts. Carefully designed writing exercises can assist in illustrating and emphasizing important ideas, and can help students "connect" with concepts through immediate application of new information. With increasing complexity, writing exercises can require more sophisticated and higher level thinking. Exercises should be designed to encourage the student to think in abstraction and to conceptualize, elaborate, generalize, interpret, and reason. All of these lead to critical thinking (Pond, Bradshaw, & Turner, 1991).

Successful writing activities require that the instructor use appropriate questioning skills to direct writing exercises in order to challenge students and stimulate thought. This requires planning and forethought, and should be an integral part of the course, rather than an "add-on" or an afterthought. Examples of questions that can be used to structure short writing exercises include:

- **Action questions**
  What can you do to facilitate return of bowel sounds in this situation?
- **Challenge questions**
  How much pain medication will you administer at this time? Why?
- **Diagnostic questions**
  What conclusions can you draw from this laboratory work?
- **Questions on priority**
  What will you do first in this situation?
- **Questions of extension**
  What are the possible consequences of this action?
- **Questions of generalization**
  In general, what are the presenting symptoms of acute MI?

In a small classroom situation, these questions are appropriate for group discussion. In larger classes, they are more effectively used as writing cues. When responded to by individual students, they have additional value as the students evaluate their own answers. Acting as a role model once the short writing exercise is done, the instructor can explain possible answers and various ways of evaluating answers, essentially demonstrating critical thinking and the process of open minded inquiry and examination of assumptions.

Learning to think critically *is a process* rather than an event, and this process takes continued practice. It must be nurtured and developed over a period of time, much as clinical expertise is developed. Indeed, the ability to think critically will ultimately be the most important skill in any nurse's repertoire. One way to make sure the student practices is to work several writing exercises (writing interludes) into each class session. Short structured questions can be combined with other methods such as admit slips, unsent letters, and buddy exchange (see Chapter Three) to elicit thinking on several different levels. These interludes can be recorded on a separate sheet and turned in at the end of class, or they can be a part of the student's notes to keep and refer back to as students review the day's proceedings.

COURSE ADMINISTRATION

Incorporating writing-to-learn strategies into a course can actually be as exciting and beneficial to the instructor as it is to the student. Especially for faculty who teach large sections, it affords the opportunity for personal communication which would not have otherwise been possible. Imagine having one-to-one contact with 160 students on a weekly basis! Using writing-to-learn strategies, this is possible.

The most important thing to remember when contemplating using these strategies is that the course should be writing intense *for the students,* not the instructor. Without careful planning, it can easily increase an instructor's workload by many hours each week. This can undermine the whole idea of writing-to-learn. It is possible to implement this and actually shift the majority of work being done in the course from the instructor to the student. Before this can happen, both faculty and student must let go of some of their traditional expectations.

Faculty and students must get accustomed to the idea that all written work does not have to be graded. Faculty can evaluate the writing and stay "in touch" with students by collecting the writing exercises at the end of class and scanning through them. It is possible to scan through 85 to 90 in less than an hour. It is not necessary to give written feedback unless the situation demands it. A great deal of information can be derived from this practice. The instructor will be able to tailor future class sessions to particular needs identified by scanning the exercises. It is also a good way to obtain ongoing evaluation of instruction. Finally, collecting written exercises in this manner can be a way to obtain an accurate class roll for the day (and avoid the age old practice of students signing the roll for their absent peers).

Another way to handle evaluation of the written exercises is to have students keep their writings in a portfolio that can be handed in at the end of the semester. Again, these portfolios do not have to be graded in the traditional sense. One very effective method is to have students evaluate the content of their own portfolios against a set of criteria, using examples to explain and illustrate the assessment of their own work. The instructor then grades the student's evaluation rather than the entire portfolio, referring to the portfolio only when needed.

Despite the effort at a paradigm shift regarding writing for a grade versus writing for the sake of writing, faculty who have implemented these strategies have consistently encountered one issue: Students want at least some kind of credit for their work. It seems students perceive that the work is somehow of less value if there is not some kind of credit attached. One way to handle this is to award participation credit for the writing exercises. In other words, if students do the writing exercise, they automatically get participation credit for that day, which is calculated into a participation component of the semester grade for the course. In this way, there is at least some recognition of the writing effort, without adding the enormous burden of grading 150 papers each week.

Another traditional belief that must be dealt with is the immediate, negative response that many students have when they hear the word "write." It immediately conjures of visions of term papers, research, and struggling to put down on paper what the student believes the professor wants. This issue must be addressed from the first minute of class. It takes explaining and re-explaining because most students are not accustomed to writing in this manner. It is helpful to have the writing-to-learn component of the course clearly spelled out in written form, in addition to verbal explanation. This may be incorporated into the course syllabus. It may also be incorporated into student/instructor contracts (Figure 14.1). This contract can be tailored to meet the needs of any class situation. While these contracts seem rather formal and structured at first glance, it is important to recognize that critical thinkers do not evolve from vagueness and ambiguity. Critical thinking evolves from discipline, structure, and repetition (Paul, 1990). The clarity of students' thinking and writing will be directly affected by the clarity of course leadership.

Figure 14.1
Student Course Contract
(Sample)

---

1. I understand that I am responsible for my own learning and that I must participate actively in the course.
2. I understand that there will be at least 20 short, in-class writing assignments in this course which are an integral part of the learning process.
3. I understand that my grade will be based on the following criteria:

Class participation	30%
Midterm exam	35%
Final exam	35%

4. I understand that the writing exercises in this course will be part of my participation grade.
5. I understand that I am accountable for adhering to the University's attendance policy and that my grade may be affected by more than two absences during the semester.
6. I understand that I am responsible for seeking faculty input and guidance if I become concerned about my grade at any point during the semester.

Whatever the class size or level of student, writing-to-learn strategies can be an important part of the teaching-learning process. These strategies give faculty a useful, practical tool for finally getting free of the didactic, content driven classes which have ruled education for hundreds of years and moving students toward higher, more sophisticated levels of thinking and communicating.

REFERENCES

American Association of Colleges of Nursing. (1992). *Position statement: Nursing's agenda for the 21st century.* Washington, DC: Author.

National League for Nursing. (1992). *Criteria and guidelines for the evaluation of baccalaureate and higher degree programs in nursing.* New York: Author. (Publication No. 15-2474)

Paul, R. (1990). *Critical Thinking.* Rohnert Park, CA: Center for Thinking and Moral Critique.

Pond, E., Bradshaw, M., & Turner, S. (1991). Teaching strategies for critical thinking. *Nurse Educator, 16,* 6, 18–22.

Chapter Fifteen

A WRITING-TO-LEARN STRATEGY FOR FAMILY SCIENCE EDUCATION

Janis G. Weber-Breaux, PhD, CFLE, CFCS

S tudents in family science programs in addition to learning information, must also learn to use that information. Family science educators aim to prepare students to be critical thinkers giving attention to learning that goes beyond assimilation of data. Writing-to-learn strategies encourage critical thinking (Allen, Bowers, & Diekelmann, 1989). The traditional learning-to-write paradigm assumes that the major purpose of writing is communication of what one knows. The writing-to-learn paradigm assumes that learning occurs through writing (Allen et al., 1989). Students taking a family relations course demonstrated a better understanding of course material when required to complete a writing-to-learn assignment called a "reflections" paper. The reflections paper was an analysis of the students' families.

OBJECTIVES

An expected outcome of the Child and Family Studies Degree Program at the University of Southwestern Louisiana is for students to acquire an understanding of the general philosophy and broad principles of family life education as encompassed within ten interdependent topics outlined by the National Council on Family Relations (1984): families in society; internal dynamics of families; human growth and development; human sexuality; interpersonal relationships; family resource management; parent education and guidance; family law and public policy; ethics; and family life education methodology. One of the courses that has focused on the topic of the internal dynamics of families is called family relations. Course objectives have included:

1. The students will demonstrate an understanding of family system concepts by completing a genogram, family chronology, and reflections paper.
2. The students will change inaccurate beliefs about marriage.

Writing-to-Learn

Strategy

Students enrolled in the undergraduate university course entitled family relations completed a writing-to-learn assignment that was carried out throughout the semester.

Students were asked to prepare a three- or four-generation genogram (some did more), a family chronology, and a writing-to-learn assignment of a family analysis paper entitled "Reflections." The instructor lectured on how to prepare a genogram, family chronology, and reflections paper during the first week of classes. Students were also assigned readings concerning genograms and the concepts of interest (Anderson, 1988; Herth, 1981; Lewis, 1989; McGoldrick & Gerson, 1985; Marlin, 1988; Maynard & Olson, 1987; Okiishi, 1987) and given an example of a family chronology.

The genogram has been described as a ". . . family tree that talks" (Marlin, 1988, p. 20). "A genogram is a format for drawing a family tree that records information about family members and their relationships over at least three generations" (McGoldrick & Gerson, 1985, p. 1). It uses symbols and colors to portray the family system.

A family chronology lists occurrences in the family in chronological order giving a brief description of each occurrence such as family births and deaths, marriages, separations, divorces, moves, and job changes. The genogram and the family chronology were due the week before mid-semester. Genograms were scored and returned within one week.

The writing-to-learn portion of the assignment, the family analysis reflections paper was due two weeks later. The genogram and the family chronology were used as starting points for "reflections" on the family processes in each generation.

Concepts to be addressed in the analysis were family emotional and intellectual development, implicit and explicit rules, and coping with crises (Weber-Breaux, 1993). Coping with crises analysis included how the family defined problems, resources, and active coping efforts. Analysis of resources included personal, social and family system resources (cohesion, adaptability, communication). The family analysis was scored on clarity of understanding family concepts.

EFFECTIVENESS

The family analysis assignment, a writing-to-learn strategy, has been shown to be effective in changing inaccurate beliefs about marriage (Weber-Breaux & Poirrier, 1994). The Marriage Quiz (Larson, 1988) was administered to experimental and control groups of undergraduate students who took the family relations course. Analysis of the difference in pre- and posttest scores indicated that the family analysis writing-to-learn strategy can help change inaccurate beliefs about marriage.

As can be seen by the following quotes from students, the family analysis writing-to-learn strategy is also an effective means of bridging the gap between lecture and text material and personal relevance:

> I also have more respect and admiration for some of my family members considering the hardships they were faced with. I realize how fortunate I am to be a part of such a stable and caring family. Thank you for giving me the opportunity to learn so much about my family.

> This analysis has been an inspiration to me by giving me a broad look into the positive changes that have happened in my life and the lives of my entire family.

> This analysis has done the purpose it was intended to do. I have learned more about my family's patterns, transitional figure, development, and coping abilities. I was also able to find similarities and differences between the generations.

> I learned very much about my family. Writing this paper helped me realize what kind of marriage I will have and what things I will have to work on to make my marriage better than those before me. I also learned what traits were passed down and why I may do the things I do.

> Preparing this genogram and personal history has been another step in my own growing process. It was very difficult at

times in having to relive certain memories, but the overall benefit I will have is yet to be recognized. I highly recommend it for this and other class assignments. It would also be a beneficial tool for family practitioners to use.

Writing this paper has brought me much closer to my parents and grandparents. It has made me aware of the reasons behind the actions and attitudes of some family members. It will also serve as a keepsake of things I will one day want to pass on to my children and grandchildren.

In conclusion, I have found many differences in my family background. I also better understand why my parents act the way they do. Coming from two totally different backgrounds, my mom and dad have found a common ground to raise their family. Although I do not approve of all the processes of either side, I can find ways to break certain undesirable patterns. After looking into my family history I have found that keeping a family close takes a lot of time and hard work.

This paper has really made me think about some of the negative aspects of our family which usually aren't talked about. I also thought about some old memories and was able to relive other memories of my grandparents. This paper also helped me discover a different part of my maternal grandparents. Because of them, this was a most pleasant experience.

Through this research I have learned many things about my family. I also understand more about my family by researching on their behavior and actions objectively. It has also helped me in ways of knowing how I would like to raise my children in the future. This research was very informative, perceptive and rewarding. I really enjoyed writing this paper.

I really enjoyed this project. I learned a lot from talking to my family. There were things that I wanted to hear and things that I did not want to hear. Sometimes after I talked to some members of my family, I cried when I was alone. Some of the stories that I was told made it easier to understand why some people are the way that they are.

The students' comments indicate that the main benefit may be less academically and more personally significant. Students may find the family analysis both therapeutic and cathartic.

CONCLUSION

The writing-to-learn strategy of family analysis used by some family science instructors has been shown to be effective in changing inaccurate beliefs about marriages and to encourage critical thinking about students' own families, their personal lives, and family science concepts.

Plans for future writing-to-learn assignments include assigning a family analysis that is composed of a series of weekly assignments. The effectiveness of the weekly assignments has not been empirically demonstrated. Weekly assignments would be consistent with the writing-to-learn paradigm. Future research could compare the effectiveness of family analysis as a large written project with the effectiveness of the family analysis as weekly assignments.

REFERENCES

Allen, D. G., Bowers, B., & Diekelmann, N. (1989). Writing to learn: A reconceptualization of thinking and writing in the nursing curriculum. *Journal of Nursing Education, 28,* 6–11.

Anderson, S. A. (1988). Parental stress and coping during the leaving home transition. *Family Relation, 37*(2), 160–165.

Herth, K. A. (1981). The root of it all: Genograms as a nursing assessment tool. *Journal of Gerontological Nursing, 15*(12), 32–37.

Larson, J. (1988). The marriage quiz: College students' beliefs in selected myths about marriage. *Family Relations, 37,* 3–11.

Lewis, K. G. (1989). The use of color-coded genograms in family therapy. *Journal of Marital and Family Therapy, 15*(2), 169–176.

McGoldrick, M., & Gerson, R. (1985). Constructing genograms. *Genograms in family assessment* (pp. 9–38). New York: Norton.

Marlin, E. (1988, January). If your family tree could talk. *Self,* 88–91.

Maynard, P. E., & Olson, P. H. (1987). Circumplex model of family systems: A treatment tool in family counseling. *Journal of Counseling and Development, 65,* 502–504.

National Council on Family Relations. (1984). *Standards and criteria for the certification of family life educators, college/university curriculum guidelines, and content guidelines for family life education: A framework for planning programs over the life span.* St. Paul, MN: Author.

Okiishi, R. W. (1987). The genogram as a tool in career counseling. *Journal of Counseling and Development, 66,* 139–143.

Weber-Breaux, J. G. (1993). The family transmission process. In M. J. Sporakowski (Ed.), *Family life education teacher's kit* (pp. 119–121). Minneapolis, MN: National Council on Family Relations.

Weber-Breaux, J. G., & Poirrier, G. P. (1994). Family analysis: Effectiveness of a writing strategy in family science learning. *Family Science Review, 7*(3–4), 105–112.

Chapter Sixteen

WRITING-TO-LEARN THE IMPORTANCE OF NURSING'S ROLE IN INFLUENCING HEALTH POLICY

Rosemary Rhodes, DNS, RN
Stephanie D. Wiggins, DNS, RN

*L*egislative action is and will continue to be a very important component in the evolution of nursing. Because many of the issues facing nursing today will be determined in the political arena, nurses must know, or come to know better, the appropriate strategies for working with legislators at the local, state, and national levels (Skaggs, 1994).

With the changes in health care occurring so rapidly, it is imperative that nurses realize their role in influencing and affecting these changes. And to do so, we turn to nursing education, the logical forum for establishing an understanding of how public policy influences nursing practice. Faculty role modeling and the nursing curricula are two significant resources for imparting to students the importance of health policy and how to participate actively in the formulation of policy.

In general, nurses need to learn how to interact, and how to interact better, with representatives in the political process. Personal contact with legislators can have an influence on the outcome of certain bills of importance to nursing and to the individual (Alabama State Nurses' Association, 1991). Nursing students have an opportunity, as representatives of the nursing community and as citizens, to establish continuous, effective communication with lawmakers. In this chapter, then, we will describe specific writing-to-learn health policy activities in a senior level nursing issues and leadership course for nursing students in a baccalaureate program that attends to such opportunities and needs.

At the University of South Alabama College of Nursing, students are introduced to health policy at the very beginning of their undergraduate education and related clinical perspectives are incorporated as students progress through the curriculum. In the senior nursing issues and leadership course, health policy is integrated from the first day of class throughout the course. The course is designed to be an empowering process. The objectives specific to this writing-to-learn activity are:

- Discriminate roles of the nurse advocate in multiple health care settings, identifying related issues, ethical dilemmas, and legal ramifications.
- Evaluate leadership roles for nurse participation in political systems and in professional nursing organizations.

Content about health policy and politics are interwoven into lectures, discussions, and written assignments in relation to issues of change, communication, conflict resolution, decision-making, influence, leadership, management, and power. The essence of politics is based on policy development and implementation skills, which encompass each of these topics just mentioned (Leavitt, 1994). As a result, this course provides the techniques needed for the student to analyze, synthesize, evaluate, and assume an active role in shaping health policy.

Writing-to-learn activities about health policy and the political process, both specifically and generally, also enable students to affect change in the clinical area at the community, state, and national level. Problems identified in the clinical area are discussed from a political and policy perspective. Students are required to report in each class a current national, state, or local news article regarding an ethical, legal, or legislative issue that influences healthcare. Information sources are diverse: newspaper articles, journal essays, newsletters, the Internet, and so on. Within each class, one hour is usually spent discussing the various issues and what the students, soon to be nurses, can do to realize their aims in the political arena.

One course assignment in particular merits consideration here, and which can be met only after careful review of current issues. The student is required to write a letter to their congressman or state legislator expressing their views about an issue. Not surprisingly, many letters have been written as a result of class discussions about current issues affecting healthcare. Students are also encouraged to make other contacts with key people explaining the issue of interest and what it means to citizens of the state and community. They may choose to visit elected officials, write letters to local newspapers, and involve others in health-related fields to advocate for consumers.

The Importance of Nursing's Role in Health Policy

To provide structure for the student and to reduce anxiety, sample letters are given to each student and the components of a letter are reviewed on the first day of class. The importance of communicating effectively with people is discussed in reference to letters and other forms of communication with legislators. This particular writing exercise, which both enlightens and animates the student, requires an in-depth knowledge of the particular issue and an analysis and synthesis of materials gathered regarding the issue. Students then formulate their letters expressing personal opinions relative to the specific health policy issue.

The lecture content itself accentuates how very important it is that nurses recognize their responsibility to participate in governmental decision making that directly and indirectly affects healthcare and thus their own future. Emphasis is placed on the importance of students being knowledgeable of proposed legislation to determine the effect issues may have on nurses as individuals and on nursing as a profession. Various resources available through the American Nurses Association, N-PAC, and legislative publications which can enhance awareness of political issues in healthcare are discussed. In addition, to facilitate an understanding of the forces driving healthcare and survival within the system, discussion of how legislative issues can and do effect organizational structure within the health care delivery system is incorporated into class content. The energetic learning atmosphere that is created by class discussion of health issues is also quite attractive to students, with resulting positive evaluations of the writing-to-learn activity. Students have openly expressed gratitude for the opportunity the class has given them to actively influence health policy development. One student commented, "For the first time I feel confident and knowledgeable enough about my concerns on health issues to really want to write my Congressman." Another student put it this way: "Until this class I never could have told you my Congressman's or any other elected official's name." Students have also expressed that they have a greater understanding of how to be involved at the local, state, and national level.

University of South Alabama nursing faculty believe now more than ever before that the writing-to-learn activity offers a style of teaching that helps to increase the self-esteem of the soon-to-be graduate. According to alumni reports, and as a result of seeds planted firmly in courses which use writing-to-learn, many of our graduates have become active in the political arena of nursing and other healthcare organizations. Certainly this experience provides all the students with the long-term skills needed to remain politically active throughout their career.

REFERENCES

Alabama State Nurses' Association. (1991). *CLOUT ASNA legislative manual* (7th ed.). Montgomery, AL: ASNA.

Leavitt, J. (1994). Policy and politics—A necessity for inclusion in nursing curricula: Our nursing practice depends on it! *Dean's Notes, 16*(2).

Skaggs, B. (1994). Political action in nursing. In J. Zerwekh & J. Claborn (Eds.). *Nursing today: Transition and trends* (pp. 236–256). Philadelphia: W. B. Saunders.

Chapter Seventeen

What Is WAC and How Do We Get It at Our University?

Christine Hult, PhD

Writing-across-the-curriculum (WAC) is a compelling idea that continues to appeal to teachers and administrators alike. As Cornell and Klooster (1990) point out, "the WAC movement has gained considerable support in our colleges and universities because its aims and methods seem simple: to teach students to write and to help them learn their academic subjects by asking them to write more, and for more diverse audiences" (pp. 14–15). But Cornell and Klooster also sound a note of caution; nothing is ever quite as simple as it may appear at first. They argue that, in fact, WAC is a very radical notion that requires a transformation of the academy, "WAC requires professors to be *teachers* first of all, not disciplinary specialists, scholars, or researchers" (p. 15). This transformative point of view requires both institutional and personal commitment. Administrations must be committed to supporting professors in various disciplines as they learn to teach their *students* as well as their *subjects*. Professors must continually be open to changing their methods and approaches, adopting what may seem to be a foreign agenda imposed from without. The programs, courses, and professors represented in this volume attest to the widespread commitment in higher education to this "radical" notion of writing to learn across the curriculum.

In this chapter, I will describe the process we have recently gone through at my university as we have sought to revise our general education program. Part of the process involved a close look at our writing program as it intersected with general education and with the written communication requirements for all students. This process illustrates broadly some of the issues and decisions that face administrators and faculty as they attempt to define writing experiences for students across the curriculum. It also illustrates how one school sought to more strongly institutionalize the WAC efforts that had been ongoing but sporadic.

WAC Programs That Work

What are the common denominators of writing-across-the-curriculum programs that work? Griffin (1985) outlines three important premises of successful WAC programs:

1. "Writing skills must be practiced and reinforced throughout the curriculum, otherwise they will atrophy, no matter how well they were taught in the beginning,"
2. "To write is to learn . . . we are really talking about a new way of teaching and learning, in which students listen less and learn more," and
3. "Since written discourse is central to university education, the responsibility for the quality of student writing is university-wide" (pp. 401–403).

For anyone embarking on a WAC adventure, these premises lie at the heart of the program. We were strongly influenced by these premises as we discussed our own program design.

Fulwiler and Young (1990) found many points of commonality in their investigation of WAC programs at various institutions, "Most institutions (1) articulate remarkably similar program goals: to improve student writing and learning in all content areas of the curriculum; (2) base their programs on a common core of language theorists, most often including some mix of James Britton, Don Murray, Janet Emig, and Peter Elbow; and (3) promote similar process-oriented composition pedagogy" (p. 2). They found a few points of difference "on issues such as the nature and scope of faculty training programs; which curricular structures best insure that program goals are met; and sources of new or continued funding" (p. 2). In the description of Utah State University's new general education program that follows, you will see how closely we mirror the WAC programs described by Fulwiler and Young.

THE DESIGN

As we thought about revising the university's written communication requirement, we strove to articulate for ourselves and for the campus community what we felt was working well about the writing program and what changes we (English department writing faculty) thought should be implemented through the general education reform. The current general education writing requirement mandates six quarter hours of writing: English 101 (Composition) and English 200 or 201 (Persuasive Writing or Research Writing). Many departments also required of their majors a third tier writing course. To serve this requirement, the English department offered multiple sections of English 301 (Advanced Writing) and English 305 (Technical/Professional Writing) each term. A few departments or colleges had also developed their own WAC programs (see, for example, the description of USU's WAC program in Civil and Environmental Engineering by Manuel-Dupont, 1996; or a description of the college of Humanities Arts and Social Sciences Rhetoric Associates program by Kinkead, 1993). These efforts were important and commendable because they laid the groundwork for future discussions of WAC on campus.

Representatives from the English faculty served on the university-wide General Education Review Task Force, which worked diligently for several years to develop a foundation philosophy for the general education reform, including the goals for writing requirements. A subcommittee of faculty with an interest in WAC, dubbed the "Writing Working Group," drafted a report that the General Education Review Task Force used as they designed the entire general education package. The Writing Working Group, with the help of writing specialists from English, articulated the philosophical statement and goals that we hoped would undergird the new general education writing requirement.

Philosophical Statement

1. Writing Is a Mode of Learning   The first principle draws upon James Britton's distinction between language for learning and language for informing. As writing theorists have discovered, writing in the schools has tended to over-emphasize writing for informing to the exclusion of all other uses of writing. Utah State's writing program must emphasize that writing is critical to idea formulation and independent thinking. It should give students experience "rendering" experience as well as explaining or analyzing it. Expressive writing helps students understand their own experiences; transactional writing helps them to communicate their experiences to others. Both functions of writing need to interact in a writing program wherein teachers provide opportunities for students to operate in both spheres. Such interaction encourages students to make use of the discovery function of writing—to write what they know in order to know what they mean.

Specific Program Goals:

1. Students will have experience with expressive writing, using reading and writing to learn about themselves and their world and to promote humanistic values and ethical approaches to communicating;

2. Students will have experience with transactional writing: learning common college-level expectations for writing, gaining exposure to a college library's resources and processes, practicing various conventional ways to organize and develop exposition, writing to present the results of critical reading, writing arguments based on analysis, using some standard form of documentation. These experiences will include in-depth understanding of the need and ethics of documentation and the philosophical and legal ramifications of plagiarism;

3. Students will have experience using the technologies of written communication, including word processing for document presentation and design, and computer searching for information access.

2. Writing Is a Complex Developmental Process The second principle addresses the problem schools have had with overemphasizing the completed writing product to the exclusion of the writing process. Writing researchers over the past twenty years or so have encouraged writing teachers to shift their focus from product to process in an effort to emphasize the importance of writing for discovery. The actual composition stage of writing follows the discovery stage in which expressive language, both oral and written, plays an important role. In expressive beginnings (classroom discussion, invention exercises, interpretive note-taking, journal writing, drafting, etc.), the writer explains the matter to him- or herself so that the explanation can be communicated to others. Furthermore, writing ability is a long-term developmental process integrally connected with cognitive growth and language skills in general, including reading skills. Utah State's new writing program, with its vertical sequence, acknowledges and parallels this complex developmental process, moving students toward cognitive growth in each subsequent writing course.

Specific Program Goals:

1. Students will have experience with a variety of processes through creating ungraded exploratory writing, creating multiple drafts of some pieces of writing, rewriting to clarify, and editing to correct their own work;

2. Students will have experience with critical reading and with analysis of readings for logic, coherence, and completeness in order to develop their own evaluative criteria appropriate for judging specific pieces of writing in specific contexts;

3. Through guided practice, students will have experience with controlling diction, style, and mechanics of writing to meet the expectations of professional readers. Students will have experience with the conventional uses of standard edited English in writing, but will at the same time learn to value their own spoken and written dialects of English.

3. Writing Embraces Discourse with Varying Purposes and Audiences The third principle addresses the need for students to become flexible in their own approaches to writing tasks. Many writing theorists have discussed the differences between discourse communities across disciplines and have noted the important social and political components to writing. Although theorists have divided discourse somewhat differently, their divisions all are related to (a) the distance between writer and audience, and (b) levels of abstraction. Both parameters demand that a writer adapt his or her writing style to the writing task. Writers need to learn to recognize and control the rhetorical effects of their language choices—to be able to discuss options and understand how to select among them given the constraints of the writing task. The writing program in Utah State's general education program needs to foster flexibility in students by allowing them opportunities for writing with a variety of aims, modes, and target audiences in writing assignments.

Specific Program Goals:

1. Students will have experience communicating information effectively to particular audiences for particular purposes. Through a variety of writing tasks, students will have experience adapting their writing for a prospective audience's needs. Students will also have experience with a variety of writing purposes, including expressive purposes, to gain the understanding that an author's purpose may be accomplished in a number of different ways;

2. Students will have experience with a range of academic writing tasks, including summaries, reports, research papers, and essay examinations. They will have experience responding, reflecting, reporting, synthesizing, and analyzing their own and others' work;

3. Students will have experience with working collaboratively. They should be shown how to help others make their writing better, as well as how to be more effective participants in group writing situations. In addition, students will experience insights about their own writing by reading and responding to others' writing.

THE NEW GENERAL EDUCATION
PROGRAM AT UTAH STATE UNIVERSITY

As the various committees worked on the general education design, the philosophical stance outlined by the Writing Working Group continued to play an important role in decision making. The new General Education program, called "University Studies" includes the following "competencies." Notice how the language and goals outlined by the Writing Working Group have now become solidified into competencies that the university desires to instill into all of its students. The five general competencies are (a) reading, listening, and viewing for comprehension, (b) communicating effectively for various purposes and audiences, (c) understanding and applying mathematics and other quantitative reasoning techniques, (d) using various technologies competently, and (e) working effectively both collaboratively and individually.

The second competency, communication, incorporates both verbal and written communication. The following description is quoted from the University Studies Objectives:

Communicating Effectively for
Various Purposes and Audiences

Communication includes speaking, listening, performing, and writing. People must deal with oral language and also with meanings carried in sign, gesture, and facial expression. The educated person also participates in technological communications. Course work supporting these attributes should enable students to:

1. Communicate effectively to a range of audiences for a variety of purposes;

2. Understand and make thoughtful use of the forms and features of language that vary within and across different contexts and cultural communities;

3. Become competent users of Global English;

4. Compare English with other languages;

5. Use a range of artistic and technological forms of communication to present ideas;

6. Engage productively, responsibly, and thoughtfully in oral communications.

Writing includes composing with words, supported by various technological, artistic, and symbolic forms. Courses in general education help students to:

1. Use a variety of sources of knowledge to inform their writing;

2. Understand the formal conventions of writing;

3. Understand and use criteria for effective writing;

4. Write for a variety of purposes;

5. Learn writers' ethical responsibilities in selecting and presenting information and ideas;

6. Use writing as a tool for learning;

7. Effectively use of text, drawing, graphs, diagrams, photographs, videos, and computer-generated graphics. (Utah State University, 1996)

THE WRITING PROGRAM AND ITS WAC COMPONENT

Given the outlined philosophy, goals, and competencies, how does the new written communication requirement at Utah State finally look? Through a lengthy process of give and take with various administrators, committees, colleges, and faculty groups, a three-tiered writing requirement was crafted as a component of the general education reform.

First Tier: English Composition (3 *semester* hours at the first-year level).

Second Tier: Research Writing (3 *semester* hours at the sophomore level).

Third Tier: Two three-hour writing intensive courses at the upper-division level.

Departments will be asked to recommend courses as writing intensive by submitting course syllabi. The initial evaluation will be by the faculty Communications Literacy Committee. The final decision will be made by the General Education Subcommittee and the Educational Policies Committee. It is hoped that through this lengthy approval process, courses that become writing intensive will be well-thought out and carefully coordinated across disciplines.

The writing faculty in the English department were extremely gratified that the six quarter hours of written communications were not only retained, but expanded to six semester hours. The new general education program is scheduled for implementation in concert with a switch from quarters to semesters at Utah State in 1998. Furthermore, we are excited about moving the upper-division writing courses to the disciplines, where we think the best instruction for students can take place. The Advanced Writing (English 301) and the Technical/Professional Writing (English 305), although marginally useful, were less than ideal because they were so generic. Under the new scheme, English 301 and 305 will be dropped and third-tier writing intensive courses will be designed by colleges and departments to more appropriately meet the needs of their own student populations, much as is described in several other chapters in this volume.

The Future of WAC at Utah State University

We are excited about the general education reform at Utah State University. But, at the same time, we are cautiously optimistic. We know that there is much more needed to maintain a healthy WAC program than simply a General Education mandate to develop writing intensive courses (Fulwiler & Young, 1990; McLeod & Soven, 1992; White, 1989; Young & Fulwiler, 1986). Fulwiler and Young (1990) outline the questions most frequently asked by administrators and developers of WAC programs. Some of these questions have been addressed by our general education reform, but others have not. To date, we have addressed the following questions:

Should writing be required in the curriculum?

What kinds of writing should be required?

What are the goals and objectives of successful WAC programs?

But we have scarcely begun to address the other equally important questions outlined by Fulwiler and Young:

What faculty training models have proved most effective?

Does WAC also work in secondary, middle, and elementary schools? If so, how do college programs articulate with them?

What are the characteristics of second-generation programs?

What is the role of the English department in WAC programs?

What kind of influence do WAC programs have on the total undergraduate curriculum?

How are programs funded? How can WAC programs be evaluated?

These important questions, and others that I'm certain will crop up along the way, must be carefully addressed by faculty and administrators as we seek to implement our new general education program and its WAC component. Of particular concern are the funding, leadership, and faculty training issues that have not been resolved on our campus. Right now, there are no plans for additional funding to implement the WAC writing-intensive courses. This is a grave oversight. We need to have a senior writing faculty member in the role of WAC Director. As White (1989) observes, "such writing courses [writing intensive upper-division courses] ought to involve faculty from all disciplines, working together under coordination from a professional in the field of writing" (p. 146).

Faculty who have been trained as teachers of writing-intensive courses are often "missionaries" for writing as a mode of learning. As White observes, "since faculty from all disciplines will necessarily be involved in teaching, they form a natural constituency for a writing-across-the-curriculum faculty development program, with all of its positive influence" (p. 146). These same faculty, however, learn very quickly that there are significant workload issues involved in teaching writing-intensive courses. "A history faculty member on my campus argues that he works twice as many hours to teach a social science expository writing class as he does to teach a history class" (p. 148). This is a legitimate faculty concern; we need to come to grips with funding issues so that we will be able to help faculty to teach WAC classes effectively without becoming burned out, whether this means reducing that faculty member's course load, lowering the number of students in writing-intensive courses, assigning teaching assistants or peer tutors, or providing additional compensation for writing-intensive courses.

Furthermore, as White also points out, faculty need to be trained to teach writing effectively in their disciplines. This training course may be in the form of seminars, guest lecturers, workshops, and so on. "Whatever plan is used, some kind of systematic and collegial seminar is necessary for a writing program to take hold" (p. 149). We need to take a hard look at how faculty are brought into the writing intensive program and how they are taught to effectively use writing to enhance student learning. "When this kind of faculty development is integrated naturally into the overall campus writing program, the campus climate for writing becomes exceedingly healthy" (White, 1989, p. 149).

Transforming the academy comes at a considerable expense of time, effort, and money. Instituting WAC on a campus cannot be done on the cheap, if it is truly to take roots and grow. "WAC brings the structural conflicts of the academy to the forefront because the teaching of writing requires instructors and administrators to place the good of the students before all else" (Cornell & Klooster, 1990, p. 15). When we truly place the good of the students first, WAC has at least a fighting chance to succeed.

REFERENCES

Cornell, C., & Klooster, D. (1990). Writing across the curriculum: Transforming the academy? *WPA: Writing Program Administration, 14*(1–2), 7–16.

Fulwiler, T., & Young, A. (1990). *Programs that work: Models and methods for writing across the curriculum.* Portsmouth, NH: Boynton/Cook.

Griffin, C. W. (1985). Programs for writing across the curriculum: A report. *College Composition and Communication, 36*(4), 398–403.

Kinkead, J. A. (1993). Taking tutoring on the road: Utah State University's Rhetoric Associates Program. In J. Kinkead & J. Harris (Eds.), *Writing centers in context* (pp. 210–215). Urbana, IL: National Council of Teachers of English.

Manuel-Dupont, S. (1996, January). Writing-across-the-curriculum in an engineering program. *Journal of Engineering Education,* 35–40.

McLeod, S. H., & Soven, M. (1992). *Writing across the curriculum: A guide to developing programs.* Newbury Park: Sage.

Utah State University. (1996). *University Studies Objectives: The Citizen Scholar.* USU General Education Document. Logan, UT: Author.

White, E. M. (1989). *Developing successful college writing programs.* San Francisco: Jossey-Bass.

Young, A., & Fulwiler, T. (1986). *Writing across the disciplines: Research into practice.* Upper Montclair, NJ: Boynton/Cook.

Chapter Eighteen

IMPROVING TEACHING, IMPROVING LEARNING

EFFECTIVELY USING WRITING-TO-LEARN ACROSS DISCIPLINES

Susan Gardner, PhD

*T*he need for graduates who can communicate effectively has increased the pressure to incorporate more writing into every course. Teachers are often reluctant to increase the number of formal writing assignments because they would potentially sacrifice course content, overwhelm themselves in paper grading, and other concerns that surface when teachers are surveyed.

The use of writing as a tool to aid learning of course material provides a means of incorporating more writing into already crowded courses. This chapter describes the use of writing-to-learn techniques in a variety of courses across the curriculum, and summarizes additional benefits that help improve teaching and learning.

No matter what discipline a person teaches, an overwhelming call in every field presently is for graduates with better communication skills (Allen, Bowers, & Diekelmann, 1989; De Simone, 1994; Scofield & Combes, 1993; Stocks, Stoddard, & Waters, 1994; Taylor & Paine, 1993). Graduates entering the workforce find writing a major function of their jobs, and much of the writing needs to be fluid, concise, precise English, not simply jargon-laden writing of the field. Graduates also need to be able to confidently write varied types of communication, everything from charts and diagnostic reports to memoranda, executive summaries, and recommendations.

Although undergraduates typically take writing courses at the beginning of their college years taught through English departments, the current trend is to incorporate more writing into all courses in the disciplines (Beall, 1991; Hafen, 1994). Hence, students do not have to take separate, additional writing classes outside their fields. The push to include more writing puts pressure on teachers to strengthen their own writing skills and knowledge of teaching writing as well as to make room for it in their courses. Too often the interpretation of including more writing in existing classes takes one form—adding another formal, polished term paper or project. These assignments take a great deal of time for students to complete and for teachers to evaluate.

Formal writing is time consuming, but it also is often narrow in scope. Professors worry about sacrificing content coverage to the need for longer, more formal writing assignments.

Ironically, including more writing in a course could improve both teaching and learning when writing is used as a *tool* for learning.

Concerns about Incorporating More Writing

In his recent book *Engaging Ideas: The Professor's Guide to Integrating Writing, Critical Thinking, and Active Learning in the Classroom,* John C. Bean (1996) identifies a major problem with how teachers across the curriculum see writing. Many teachers associate "good writing primarily with grammatical accuracy and correctness and thus isolate writing instruction within English departments, the home of the grammar experts." This view translates "writing as a set of isolated skills" (p. 15). This view of writing—besides relegating it to the domain of English teachers—also suggests that good writers "happen" since they seem to effortlessly produce eloquent texts, and less apt writers struggle to produce minimally acceptable prose because they lack the right "set of isolated skills."

This view of writing as seamless and linear for good writers is incorrect. A second misunderstanding involves the view of what constitutes "real writing" (Moore, 1994). Since most writing instruction takes place in English courses, students, who later turn into professors, come to view this as the only valid form of "real writing." Writing appropriate to English or humanities courses—the personal narrative, the theme on literature analysis, the argumentative essay, the documented term paper—is often not the best assignment for computer science, nursing, biology, or business students.

Concerns about using more writing are legitimate. It is not uncommon for teachers in professional areas to feel overwhelmed by the fast-changing content in their fields. They already struggle with keeping up or quickly learning new content, techniques, or technology and then turning around and teaching these areas in their classes. They might also struggle with emotional and psychological baggage left over from their own experiences with writing instruction. They often feel inadequately prepared to teach writing to students. In addition, many teachers are uncomfortable evaluating writing since it requires making subjective judgments, a judgment they feel is out of their area of expertise. They may also fear that grading writing assignments could easily bury them in mountains of papers (Stocks, Stoddard, & Waters, 1992).

Probably the most pervasive concern, however, is that time covering the discipline's body of knowledge—the content—will have to be sacrificed to provide writing instruction for more formal, finished projects and reports. Not as many pages of text, nor problems, nor concepts can be covered if students are going to be asked to write more papers.

Bean (1996), however, contends that the notion of reducing content coverage is a major misconception. He suggests that "emphasizing writing and critical thinking in a course increases the amount of subject matter that students actually learn and in many cases can actually increase *total coverage of content*" (p. 9). Other researchers (Black, 1994; Jewett, 1991; Liss & Hanson, 1993) concur. What changes to make the increase possible are two things: the teacher's role and the students' responsibility. By incorporating the technique of using writing as a tool for learning, called *writing-to-learn*, students read their texts more thoughtfully and understand material better. Teachers, then, shift from being the readers and explainers of content and assignments to facilitating and coordinating students' learning.

Writing-to-Learn—What It Is, How It Works

Simply put, *writing-to-learn* is the use of writing to help a person understand or make sense of information, learn a new concept, or move forward on a project. It is writing done to make material one's own or to grapple with difficult content. The format or style of the writing is left up to the writer. Some writers make short lists, use notecards, or scribble on double entry pages. Some of the writing takes the form of full sentences or paragraphs. Some people find doing full-pages of free or journal writing the most helpful. Others use diagramming or flow charts, graphing, or schematics to help make sense of content. Whatever feels comfortable to the writer and gets the job done is acceptable in the context of using writing to learn.

For students, writing-to-learn activities provide continuous writing practice in a nonthreatening environment. This type of writing is meant to be exploratory and not polished. As Britton and his colleagues (1975, pp. 11–18) noted over twenty years ago, informal, exploratory writing taps into a student's expressive mode of thinking and writing. Expressive writing—close to the self, engaged, exploratory—has links to higher order or critical thinking in its earliest state. It is thinking in process, still forming, and in search of clarity. Allen et al. (1989) note how important it is to shift students from their intense concentration on the finished product to the process of writing and thinking at work. Short, in-class writing-to-learn exercises aid in getting ideas down quickly or organizing thoughts rapidly as they occur. This type of writing emphasizes content first, and, if the writing is headed toward a finished product, these quick drafts may form some of the material found in the later, polished pieces. At the very least, writing-to-learn exercises provide a forum for idea generation and practice in fluency, valuable for all writers, and especially valuable for writers where English is a second language.

For teachers, writing-to-learn answers many of the fears about incorporating more writing into their courses. Writing-to-learn activities are easy to use in any discipline, and they increase the amount of writing in a course without having to introduce additional formal writing assignments. Informal in style and format, they can be done spontaneously by the instructor, take no special training in writing instruction, nor should they increase paper grading. Since this writing is primarily for students' thinking, the activities are often not collected, and those that are collected are generally not graded. A quick reading and simple check mark to indicate the exercise was recorded are enough.

WRITING-TO-LEARN ACTIVITIES IN PRACTICE

In interdisciplinary workshops on writing-to-learn, colleagues at Westminster College of Salt Lake City discussed and briefly practiced the use of this technique for incorporating more writing into their classes. Writing-to-learn activities can be classified into two major types—longer, sustained assignments and short, in-class uses. Although their exercises and purposes varied, professors subsequently reported that the writing-to-learn activities "worked just like you said they would!" Additional benefits took them by surprise.

Sustained Writing-to-Learn Assignments

Computer Science   A computer-science teacher has experimented with journals in a number of upper division courses. In computers and society and a condensed parallel programming course, she had students keep journals to record their thinking about assigned reading and ethical issues discussed in class. In operating systems and a computer architecture class, her students used the journal as a forum for writing and thinking about the course content, the assigned text, and outside reading the teacher provided. The professor felt the use of this sustained writing-to-learn activity encouraged more communication from her often taciturn students. The journals greatly increased their opportunities for writing practice, something she felt the computer science curriculum generally lacks.

Accounting   One professor used a journal in his Intermediate Accounting course for a number of reasons. One was his desire to provide writing practice and to increase writing fluency in a major which, like computer science, students often do not associate with a great deal of writing. A practicing accountant, by contrast, does a lot of writing—to clients, to the IRS, to colleagues—and in a variety of forms—letters, memoranda, detailed footnotes, reports and briefs, and so on, and accounting majors need the writing practice. His own difficult experience with college writing teachers made him fear and avoid writing, and this held-over baggage is another reason he wants accounting students to become comfortable with writing. Hence, his assignment to keep a journal over two semesters fills a need he sees as critical in the development of a competent accountant.

In his journal assignment, the professor asks students to respond to readings, to class discussions, to hypothetical cases, to test questions, to how the class is going, and so on. Some of the writings are focused by his explicit directions; others he leaves open-ended for students' own choice. Increased student-teacher communication is a natural by product of the writing and response activity of a journal, and this professor believes the writing practice in the first semester in the non-threatening environment of a journal helps students make the transition in the second semester to more formal writing assignments modeled on actual accounting situations.

Science   Although writing-to-learn may not be the label science professors have used to denote their science or field notebook assignments, this type of writing is an excellent example of the sustained use of the technique for learning content. In an integrated, introductory science course for nonscience majors team-taught by physics, biology, and chemistry professors, the double-entry science notebook is a major component for learning. This course, sponsored by the National Science Foundation, is lab-based and makes use of writing as scientists do—to record data and observations, describe lab experiments and processes, draw or diagram phenomena, do simple calculations, and so on.

In addition to writing a kind of factual account of "doing science," reflective writing is also used as the second entry in the notebook. This reflective writing sets the context of a lab by first summarizing what students are working on and what contributions that work makes to their science knowledge up to that point. Reflective entries also make connections to assigned reading, personal knowledge, or reading and experiences outside of class. These entries are also places to wonder and ask the "what if . . ." and "how do . . ." questions about the natural world.

Literature   In an introductory literature course, an English professor regularly required students to write and turn in a "reader response" to the assignment before the reading was discussed in class. By end of the term, students needed to have 25 full pages of responses to the 40 plus reading assignments. The responses could range from a quandary of "I don't understand anything this author is saying" to a discussion of a particular metaphor or symbol a poet used. All that was required was an honest response, a full-page or 15-minute write after an initial reading, and a total of 25 pages by term's end. Teaching assistants and the teacher made minimal comments to the 52 students' writes and recorded their completion as they were turned in. When the professor suggested in the course evaluation doing away with this requirement, students' protests were overwhelming. Many students had exceeded the required number of pages because writing with reading was so helpful to their understanding. In addition, over a third of the class responded that the reader responses gave them a method to keep current with assignments and forced them to really grapple with the content. The professor decided to keep the requirement in future literature courses.

Short Writing-to-Learn Exercises

Shorter writing-to-learn activities can be done at the beginning, in the middle, or at the end of classes and, again, for a variety of purposes. For example, a 5- to 10-minute assignment during class can help students prepare more effectively for group work or class discussions or serve as springboards to get them started on longer assignments or projects. Several professors have used brief writes to break the pace of a class period by having students react to the lecture, ask their own questions, respond to a specific prompt, define terms, make connections, and so on.

Nursing   Although writing short responses to research articles or descriptions of clinical practices are typical of writing-to-learn exercises in a nursing program, some lighter activities in an intense curriculum can be used. For example, one nursing professor used short, in-class assignments to help introduce students to each other and generally establish the importance of community building for the class. After briefly describing the course and introducing herself, the professor asked students to write the answer to a simple sentence stem, "I think I'm the only one in the room that . . . ." Following a few minutes of thinking and writing, students went around the room, stated their names, and read their sentences aloud. A simple technique helped ease the tensions of starting a new and highly competitive program, and the teacher continued to use writing-to-learn techniques throughout the course to monitor progress, build community, and evaluate where students were in their conceptual thinking.

Management   A professor in the MBA program had students write a list of five major organizational concepts the class had been studying and then briefly describe how those five areas related to the company they worked for. Following this private brainstorming session, students were grouped together to share their lists and discuss how they were going to approach their semester project. The professor was amazed at how productive the small groups were after having taken a brief time to write first. He noted that the individual writing and the peer group discussion enabled each student to determine if he or she had five concepts down accurately and if each was making appropriate connections to the workplace. In this case, then, the writing-to-learn activity enabled a number of things to occur:

- Reinforcement of course concepts.
- Quick check on understanding of the components of an assignment.
- Initial progress on topic choice and basic information for a major project.
- Commitment to five concepts and their connection to a workplace setting necessary to complete the assignment.

- Effective preparation for contributing to a small group discussion.

This activity also shifted the work from the teacher to the students. The teacher did not have to collect and read through papers to ensure that students were on track. The writing activity combined with peer group discussion served as the enablers of learning.

This same management professor, a strong advocate of writing-to-learn, has used brief writes during class for other reasons. Since he often teaches lengthy weekend or night block courses, this professor sometimes uses a brief write at the beginning of a class to clear the students' brains of "noise." A high percentage of his students are working professionals who come to class full of the day's work pressures, concerns about their families, difficulties with finances, and so on. Asking students to freewrite for 10 minutes about whatever is on their minds allows them to put their worries and distractions in concrete form and then file them until class is over. Noticing or addressing student concerns in this manner creates a more productive class, the professor believes. Somehow having made the lists or written about frustrations at work serves as a mind clearer and then students are ready to concentrate on the evening's lecture or activities.

ADDITIONAL POSSIBILITIES FOR WRITING-TO-LEARN

Several writing-to-learn activities have been suggested in the preceding section, but teachers across disciplines might think of trying some of the following possibilities to help students learn the content of the course:

- Respond to a video, guest speaker, new concept or technique.
- Restate esoteric material or a difficult problem in their own words.

- Predict or hypothesize to manipulate a problem or model.
- Write what they know about a topic before study begins and then again after working through the topic.
- Define unfamiliar terms and specialized vocabulary.
- Draw a diagram, graph, or flow chart of a process or model.
- Describe one thing they learned from the day's class.
- Summarize the main points of a lecture or a guest speaker's presentation.
- List one or two questions about a topic that needs further clarification.
- Write from an opposing viewpoint when a controversial topic is being discussed.
- Explain a discovery they made as a result of a lecture, discussion, or reading.
- Critique a reading, writing, or project assignment.
- Assess their own learning of a concept, skill, or information.
- Roughly outline the structure they are using to complete a project.
- Explain difficulties or frustrations they encounter on a project.
- Summarize the progress they are making on a long-term assignment.
- Evaluate how a class is going—level of difficulty, variety of assignments, student satisfaction, etc.
- Describe potential trouble spots in a collaborative assignment or project.
- Outline main points, methodology, and conclusion of a research article.
- Identify what they need to know yet to complete a term or research project.

The list of possibilities for using writing-to-learn activities is only limited by a teacher's imagination and students' needs for understanding in a course. These preceding suggestions are ones that teachers at several levels—elementary, secondary, and college—have tried and found useful.

BENEFITS OF Writing-to-Learn

The major benefit of writing-to-learn activities is increased active learning. Writing-to-learn is productive; that is, reading, researching, data collecting, and writing about the content significantly improves retention, understanding, and ability to use the knowledge gained (Soven, 1995). In her research, Collins (1985) notes that reading accompanied by informal, expressive writing, that is, writing for the self and not for performance, served as an aid to increase reading comprehension. When used during class, writing-to-learn activities can encourage active learning instead of the passive learning or even lack of learning that frequently occurs during lectures. Longer, sustained, out-of-class writing-to-learn assignments help students take more responsibility for their learning. To be able to write about content, they have to work their way into understanding it, and writing gives them the vehicle to do this.

Writing-to-learn activities can increase writing fluency in all students just through the practice of putting concepts and thoughts into written English. When used frequently enough, students whose first language is not English can experience marked improvement in fluency.

Real improvement in writing skills requires someone to respond to the additional areas of organization and mechanics, and writing improvement is best seen through multiple drafts of documents. Writing-to-learn activities, however, can provide a bridge to writing improvement because such practice produces the facility necessary for more formal papers. In addition, writing-to-learn activities help students who are already competent writers to maintain their skills and increase their comfort level with writing. An additional benefit is that learning to use writing as a method or tool for understanding is a lifelong skill, not one confined to formal education. On the job, at home, personally and professionally, writing can be used to solve problems.

For teachers pressed to include more writing in their content courses, writing-to-learn activities provide a practical solution to an already overcrowded curriculum. These informal, "first thinking" activities not only provide writing practice; they also allow teachers to hear all the voices in a class and provide teachers with windows into students' thinking and thinking processes. These windows, in turn, help teachers to monitor students' progress and the flow of a course, and, thus, they can react to difficulties much sooner. Having students write frequently fosters the development of critical thinking and problem solving skills, improves class discussions by holding students accountable for their reading, and shifts teachers' roles. Students who are engaged in their learning are generally more satisfied, and teachers and students both acknowledge improved student/teacher relationships as a result of this frequent, informal communication. Although it takes some sustained attention and practice to use writing-to-learn activities effectively, they can help teachers incorporate more writing into their courses in a productive and fairly painless way.

REFERENCES

Allen, D., Bowers, B., & Diekelmann, N. (1989). Writing to learn: A reconceptualization of thinking and writing in the nursing curriculum. *Journal of Nursing Education, 28*(1), 6–11.

Beall, H. (1991). In-class writing in general chemistry: A tool for increasing comprehension and communication. *Journal of Chemical Education, 68*(2), 148–149.

Bean, J. (1996). *Engaging ideas: The professor's guide to integrating writing, critical thinking, and active learning in the classroom.* San Francisco: Jossey-Bass.

Black, K. (1994). What to do when you stop lecturing: Become a guide and a resource. In S. Kadel & J. Keehner (Eds.), *Collaborative learning: A sourcebook for higher education* (Vol. 2). University Park, PA: National Center on Postsecondary Teaching, Learning, & Assessment.

Britton, J., Burgess, T., Martin, N., McLeod, A., & Rosen, H. (1975). *The development of writing abilities*. London: Macmillan Education.

Collins, C. (1985). The power of expressive writing in reading comprehension. *Language Arts, 62*(1), 48–54.

De Simone, B. (1994). Reinforcing communication skills while registered nurses simultaneously learn course content: A response to learning needs. *Journal of Professional Nursing, 10*(3), 164–176.

Hafen, M. (1994). Developing writing skills in computer science students. *ACM SIGCSE Bulletin, 26*(1), 268–270.

Jewett, J. (1991, September/October). Learning introductory physics through required writing assignments. *Journal of College Science Teaching, 20*–25.

Liss, J., & Hanson, S. (1993, May). Writing-to-learn science. *Journal of College Science Teaching, 342*–345.

Moore, R. (1994, March/April). Writing to learn biology: Let's stop neglecting the tool that works best. *Journal of College Science Teaching, 289*–295.

Scofield, B., & Combes, L. (1993). Designing and managing meaningful writing assignments. *Issues in Accounting Education, 8*(1), 71–85.

Soven, M. (1995). *Write to learn: A guide to writing across the curriculum*. Cincinnati, OH: Southwestern Publishing Co.

Stocks, K., Stoddard, T., & Waters, M. (1992). Writing in the accounting curriculum: Guidelines for professors. *Issues in Accounting Education, 7*(2), 193–204.

Taylor, H., & Paine, K. (1993). An inter-disciplinary approach to the development of writing skills in computer science students. *ACM SIGCSE Bulletin, 25*(1), 274–278.

INDEX

Index

Index

Index

Index

Index